Looking at the Stars

Looking at the Stars

Living with Cancer

Compiled and published by the

Cambridge Cancer Help Centre

Designed and edited by Tricia Smith

First published in Great Britain in 2003 by the
Cambridge Cancer Help Centre
1a Stockwell Street, Mill Road
Cambridge CB1 3ND

A CIP catalogue record for this book is available from
the British Library

ISBN 0-9545603-0-2

Typeset by Anne Clue
Fareham
Hampshire

Printed and bound in Great Britain by
Printarea Limited
Fareham
Hampshire

Dedicated to
all the brave, wonderful and inspiring people
who have visited our Centre

Illustrations

Paintings by Fiona Benham
'*Fenland Rising'*
'*Looking at the stars'*
'*Meditation'*
'*Harlequin'*
Photograph of '*Bones'* by Anne Rivington

Contents

About this book

Some years ago Ann, our Centre Co-ordinator, had one of those 'wouldn't it be wonderful if ...' moments as her head touched her pillow one night. 'Wouldn't it be wonderful if we could produce a book about our Centre that would inspire and help someone who had just received a cancer diagnosis and needed guidance on what to do and where to turn?' She talked about the idea and thought about it over the years, but nothing happened: the time was not quite right. She mentioned it to Fiona, one of the brightest in our galaxy of stars, who was enthusiastic and began to write about her own experience of cancer. But the project would probably be costly, and would also require someone with sufficient enthusiasm and determination to take it to a conclusion. So nothing happened.

But when Fiona died in September 2000, her friends and family gave the Centre a very generous donation, and the Trustees felt that it would be appropriate to use that money towards the production of 'The Book'. It was at that point that I felt sufficiently moved to volunteer to take the project forward.

For the Summer 2001 newsletter, Fiona's friend Karen wrote,

"Shortly after Fiona died last year, her friends and family decided to stay in touch with each other. We talked on the phone, wrote to each other and some of us met up trying to ease our way through the loss of our friend. We decided that we would like to do something as a group to remember her on her birthday in March.

It seems particularly fitting that we should make a contribution to the Cambridge Cancer Help Centre, since having Fiona in your life was like having your very own support group.

There are many of us who miss her special brand of nurturing and support and know how invaluable it is to have the right help and advice at critical times in your life. In just such a way the Cambridge Cancer Help Centre made a big difference to the quality of Fiona's life after her diagnosis. It gave her many new friends as well as practical, emotional and spiritual support during her illness.

This year's donation is to be spent on the writing of a book which will help people just like Fiona who have been diagnosed with cancer. We are delighted that it is going towards a book that so well reflects Fiona's spirit of optimism and practicality whilst living with cancer."

Since then Fiona's network of family and friends have met each year on her birthday, and have sent further generous donations, considerably swelling our book fund.

So we are deeply indebted to 'Fiona's Network',
which has helped to make the publication of this book possible.

Editor

Acknowledgements

I am most grateful to the many people who have supported and encouraged me throughout this project, among them the following. I hope I haven't left anyone out.

My thanks to ~

Marilyn Barnes for setting the seed in 1986

'Fiona's Network' for financial support

Brigit Viney and Nick Judd for their support at the very beginning of this venture and for their advice on publishing

Hazel Marshall for sharing her knowledge, opening my eyes to the world of publishing and introducing me to the delights of Peter Finch's book 'How to Publish Yourself'

Viv Neville and her daughter Jenny for endless typing in the early days

Fran Dawson for her meticulous proof reading and David Wilson for advice and proof reading

Anne Rivington for allowing us to reproduce the photograph of her sand sculpture

Barbara Hooper, Fiona Benham's mother for giving us permission to reproduce Fiona's paintings

Anglia Photoworks Cambridge for preparing three of Fiona's paintings for the printer

Anne Clue for so generously and conscientiously converting the text for the printer, and her friends Sue Portman and Lisa Snape for their professional help ~ without these three the whole project would have cost much more

The Repro House, Digital Impact, Waterlooville, and the Printer, Printarea, Fareham, for their perseverance in perfecting the colour graduation on the front cover

My computer-literate young friend Daniel Halford for his invaluable technical help and unwavering support and enthusiasm for the project from the beginning

Pat Pilkington and Erica Lowry for their thoughtful reviews

Karen Wolstenholme for her review and for being the mainstay of my support network, casting her critical eye on the text as it has evolved over the months, and for being the inspiration behind the colours used for the front cover

The Trustees for trusting me with this project which I've enjoyed enormously

The members of our Centre, past and present, who have written so movingly about their experiences of cancer and who have been willing to share their stories with us

And my warmest thanks to Ann Dingley for willing this book to happen, for selecting and typing much of the material and for being with me every step of the way offering encouragement and moral support.

What others are saying about this book

"In his book 'The Luck Factor' Dr Richard Wiseman says that 'lucky' people turn negative events into positively good ones. So they say 'If I hadn't broken my ankle, I wouldn't have been in the A & E department at the hospital and wouldn't have met my future husband! It was a lucky break!' In the same way 'Looking at the Stars' tells of chance encounters with healers and therapists; of deep friendships forged in the fires of cancer diagnosis; of a loving, supportive community whose joy it is to welcome, comfort and guide people in crisis.

Something quite extraordinary arises in us when we enter the crisis zone. As they say 'In crisis the soul comes to the surface' with its acute appreciation of love and beauty, of music and nature.

There is something immensely moving and uplifting in the personal stories that make up 'Looking at the Stars'. The courage, the humour, the resourcefulness, the comradeship of these wonderful people cannot fail to uplift the reader and inspire a new and enhanced way of looking at life. This little book is a tribute to the many great souls who learned how to turn negative to positive, to create pure gold out of the lead of the cancer experience. These are the modern alchemists and they have the power to show us, the readers, how to do the same. What a gift!"

Pat Pilkington   Co-founder of Bristol Cancer Help Centre

"The Cambridge Cancer Help Centre has developed a vibrancy of spirit and a breadth of resources that have touched many lives since I first came into contact with it in 1993. It is important that Centre members have had the energy to record the landmarks of this decade. They have allowed a medley of voices to tell important stories. Their accounts are sensitive and encouraging.

As a Macmillan Nurse it is my privilege to meet people who face their cancer in a variety of ways. Not all wish to join a support group. I am sure however, that many would find in 'Looking at the Stars' a resonance that could inform and support them through the turmoil and helplessness of a new cancer diagnosis. Health professionals sometimes worry that, for some, 'fighting spirit' can ultimately engender feelings of guilt and failure if they do not overcome their cancer. This book illustrates well, however, that such spirit is about exploring potential and recognising that there will be difficult times while remaining informed and in control.

The Gog Magog hills south of Cambridge provided the backdrop to my reading of 'Looking at the Stars'. I took some breaks to do my own looking and thinking. There is a sense in which one shares the emotions and stands alongside the individuals as they record their experiences. Their eloquence and insights deserve the reader's unhurried and compassionate attention. Honesty, pain, joy, humour and much wisdom are contained in this small book. It bears repeated return visits."

Erica Lowry Macmillan Clinical Nurse Specialist

"When I first visited the Cambridge Cancer Help Centre, I was impressed with the warmth of the people around me. I felt so at home that I joined in with an art therapy session. This was the first time since school that I had picked up a paintbrush. It's that kind of place.

My relationship with the Centre continued after my friend Fiona's death. I knew she had made and loved many friends there and it had been her lifeline. She had wanted people to know that there really is 'a life after cancer'. I was so proud of her and she remains a powerful inspiration in my life. Fiona knew of the plans for this book and she was so excited about it that it seemed natural for her friends and me to continue to support the project after she had gone.

I am delighted that Tricia and the Centre have now brought the book to life. This collection of personal stories and illustrations gives a powerful insight into the kaleidoscope of feelings that people have to manage if they're diagnosed with cancer. Here you will find a wealth of anecdotes describing their individual journeys, and how they made sense of what was happening to them.

This book powerfully illustrates some of the many inspirational and loving ways people come to terms with their own diagnosis. It is a journey of discovery that offers many gifts to the reader. And while it is a memorial to a few of the many wonderful people who are and have been involved with the Centre, it is also a testament to the loving people who run it. This book charts their humour, their grief, their fears and their hopes as they reconnect with health and with happiness.

These are stories about relationships ~ the connection we have with ourselves and those around us. Love, to put it simply, and the power of joining with others. Research has shown that cancer sufferers live longer if they have the love and caring support of friends. Centres such as this bridge the gap between medical needs and spiritual, mental and emotional needs. This book is a great opportunity to spread their much needed love and support to a wider audience. Long may the Centre continue its wonderful work."

Karen Wolstenholme Kinesiologist and Fiona's Network

Beginnings ~ Setting the Seed

*C*ancer changes lives: that is certain. But very often that change is as much a positive change as a negative one. If Marilyn hadn't had cancer our Centre might never have been born. So what must have been a devastating blow for her became the seed from which our Centre emerged.

After her operation, the surgeon told Marilyn that everything was looking good and that she should come back to the hospital in three months' time. 'But', she said to herself, 'what can I do to fight the cancer, to stay well, to give myself the best chance of a full recovery?'

Marilyn felt that mutual support would be beneficial. But that was in 1986 when there were very few self-help groups around. One solution, she thought, would be to form a group herself. And that is exactly what she did.

Marilyn recalls ~

*B*eginning the Cambridge Cancer Help Centre was, in large measure, my first effort at helping myself after having cancer. The support of my daughter, Sophie, was crucial. Together we decided to venture out into what was then unknown territory. I had heard of the Bristol Cancer Help Centre which was then run as a support group from someone's home, but had little idea of what happened there.

I had read everything I could find about self-help; books were few and far between on the topics we take for granted nowadays. It was my personal feeling that just being with others in a similar situation must be helpful in itself. I remember being extremely nervous on our first evening when just two people turned up. After all, I had never done anything like this before and really had no idea whether it would work. Eventually, we planned a programme, which gave everyone a chance to socialise, express themselves individually to the group if they wanted to and learn a few techniques of self-help. We always ended our two-hour meetings with relaxation.

The people who came were amazing. I learned so much from them and will always be thankful to them. The whole experience was a steep learning curve for us all. For many of us it was about learning not to be afraid in a very frightening situation. The support we gave each other was also a learning process and introduced us to the idea of giving unconditional love to people other than our family and friends. We didn't call it that then, perhaps, but that is what it was. It changed our lives because, out of our need, we learned a new way to relate to each other, and giving that kind of love to each other affects everything in our lives.

Nowadays, we all talk about these things much more openly and it is hard to remember that we were so much more inhibited then, but we were definitely aware that we had something very important in our group.

The Seed Bears Fruit

By the early 90's, Marilyn, for personal reasons, felt ready to hand over the running of the Centre. A big leap forward was made in its development when Ann Dingley became involved in 1993. Ann explains how it happened.

*M*y mum had cancer. Someone told me about 'The Bristol Programme', written by Penny Brohn, who co-founded, with Pat Pilkington, the Bristol Cancer Help Centre, and in it I read this glorious description of meditation:

"During the course of meditation you may realise that you have just returned to an awareness of your breath, but you have been away somewhere else for a while. You may not know quite what has happened to you; you were not asleep, you were not daydreaming ~ you were there, but you were not there. This is a sweetly exquisite experience that is beyond words. If it happens to you, you will know for yourself why people make such a song and dance about meditation, and you will never have to make yourself do it ever again. You will never want to stop."

That sounded very appealing to me and I contacted the Bristol Centre to ask if they knew anyone in Cambridge who taught their kind of relaxation/meditation. 'Marilyn Barnes' was their answer.

I didn't contact Marilyn immediately, but a few months later while working as a freelance trainer, I was asked to provide training cover for one week at Royal Mail. During a coffee break someone was telling me about one of the staff there named Brian. They said he had cancer. "But does he know about Marilyn Barnes?" I asked, "someone must tell him about Marilyn", I implored. So they introduced me to Brian ~ a lovely 'one-off' is what I would say about him. And he knew all about Marilyn. Through Brian I was introduced to the Cambridge Cancer Help Centre, and soon afterwards I joined the Centre's Management Committee.

It seemed the Centre's ambition was to open five days a week, well .... to buy a house and open five days a week, but house prices had risen enormously in Cambridge and the money already saved from various fund-raising activities would no longer buy a property.

One night, in bed, during the one minute or less I have between head touching pillow and falling asleep, I suddenly had this idea. What if I offered to run the Centre and we found some premises to rent.

I can't remember if I sat up in bed and wrote to Marilyn with this suggestion or whether I wrote to her first thing the next morning. I do remember that her response was very rapid. At the next Management Meeting it was discussed. To that meeting came Elizabeth Wilson, our treasurer David's wife. She had temporarily discharged herself, or at least got permission from the hospital to be at that meeting and I remember, as I met her *(I think for the first time)* thinking how wonderful and well she looked, seemingly without any cares. She gave me a hug ~ the meeting progressed ~ I left the room and the decision was taken. I became the Director of the Cambridge Cancer Help Centre.

The ball rolled quickly. I gave in my notice to the Family Health Service Authority *(as it was known then)* where I was working, and I said I didn't want them to collect for a leaving present *(because they always seemed to have to collect for someone)* but on my last day they surprised me with some money for the Centre. And the Health Authority *(as it is known now)* still asks me back to run courses occasionally.

I remember Marilyn telling me that when our Centre opened, she went to Elizabeth's bedside at the Arthur Rank Hospital, held her hand and said "Elizabeth ~ the Centre we've wanted for years has opened", and Elizabeth was very delighted.

The Centre was officially opened by the Mayor of Cambridge in temporary premises provided by Redmayne, Arnold and Harris, a local estate agent. I remember that in my 'speech' I said that we were very happy the Centre now existed and that we recognised there were many links in the chain to this success, and also that some of the links were no longer with us ~ I was thinking particularly about Elizabeth, who sadly didn't live to see that day.

Since those early days our Centre has grown
from the two who attended Marilyn's first meeting
to a membership today in excess of two hundred and fifty people.
We now open as a drop-in centre for two mornings a week,
and our telephone help line is always available.

'First-timer' Anxiety

Most of us feel a little anxious when we go somewhere on our own for the first time. And when that place is a Cancer Help Centre there's an added worry and we're not quite sure whether this is really the place for us. Olga was one such lady who several years ago knocked timidly on the wrong door and then quickly walked away when nobody answered. But just in time someone noticed she was there and ran up the road after her and brought her back. She came in trembling and bewildered, and sat nervously on the edge of her chair. After tea and biscuits she accepted a soothing hand massage and later a healing session. The ice had been broken and she became a regular visitor until her death some time ago. Since then her husband has continued to visit us and has become a very enthusiastic member of our group, raising large sums of money for our Centre from many of the pubs in the area.

Marilyn mentioned this anxiety in the Centre's first Newsletter in June 1990 when she wrote:

*M*any people feel reluctant to join a group and many have come to their first meeting at the Centre in a state of apprehension, wondering what on earth it will be like to be with other people with cancer. Fortunately, for most of us, it has been an open door to a new way of looking at life ~ and death. Simple, open-hearted interaction with others is something which is not usually achieved in normal social intercourse and it is this openness which is so healing. Meeting each other without judgement and without preconceptions, we accept each other as we are and we are able to be completely ourselves.

The good news we bring, as a group, is the knowledge that we are not alone. There is a great difference between fighting cancer as an individual without support, and fighting cancer with a supportive group of friends who are dealing with similar problems.

Notes from a new girl ~
Viv's description of her first visit to the Centre

When I arrived in Stockwell Street, I wondered what I was doing there. Wasn't enough of my time already taken up with my illness? I wouldn't know anybody and the only common factor would be illness. Depressing. And where exactly was the Centre? I was told at the corner video shop, that ~ no, they didn't know where '1a' was. I was all for giving up. No, I would just stroll up the road and see what that notice was on the church door on the other side of the road. And that's how I found the Centre.

I rang the quaint bell pull and stood outside the cherry red door and waited. Margot opened the door almost immediately. I was welcomed as though I had been expected. The outside of the building had given me no hint of the tasteful, spacious room I was to find inside. It was lovely ~ comfortable and homely ~ a room I could enjoy. Here was a feeling of freedom. Stay for the whole morning, or drop in for a while, come alone or with a friend and whatever my mood. Simply chill out or chat to new friends, leaf through a helpful book from the well-stocked shelves, benefit from healing or join in the guided meditation, put the forthcoming social events in my diary, listen to Pachelbel or .... buy half a dozen free range fresh-laid eggs and have a memorable slice of home-made apricot tart and honey and camomile tea *(my choice!)*. Relaxing! No pressure, no demands. An empathy, acceptance, and understanding. People with time. Strong, courageous, positive people. There was a shoulder to cry on, a sympathetic ear, a helping hand or simply the space to be ~ characteristics of the rapport that exists in the happiest of families.

And that was how the Cambridge Cancer Help Centre
struck me the first time I went.

Carol's experience of her first visit to the Centre

1 first went to the Centre on a day when six other new people arrived. Ann found time for us all. I have continued to go to the Centre weekly, sometimes on both days. My husband Ian usually goes with me. We have had healing and joined in with the relaxation, we drink tea, and we talk and talk and talk.

The old me would be amazed that I needed a support group. My view of myself was as a supporter *(30 years of social work)*, not someone who needed support. I soon learned. I have found the Centre to be exactly the lifeline that the title of their newsletter suggests. I find the relaxed style exactly right. Ann's unobtrusive care of us all, coupled with her unfailing ability to spot and respond to distress, is a model I admire. It sets the tone for mutual support and self-help. The continuum between those seeking support and those offering it is seamless and invisible.

The Centre is also a great source of information ~ from its library of books and tapes, and more importantly, from everyone else who attends. There is a network of people, all on their own journeys, and we share experiences and information.

I have found these contacts profoundly inspiring
and have been immensely helped
by being able to offer support as well as receive it.

Like many of our friends here at the Centre, Carol found that together with its negative effects, the cancer experience also brought with it some life-enhancing changes, and she adds:

*I*n the last few months I have also found myself on another journey ~ again rather to my surprise. I am on a spiritual journey, which has become central to my life. I have moved from a routine church attender to accepting that I am totally in God's hands. I now receive Christian Healing and my faith has developed in a way that I find exciting and wonderfully enriching. The quality of my hopefulness is now quite different.

My experiences since diagnosis have been life-changing in the extreme. I still have occasional dark days, but I never forget that I could have died some months ago. I am grateful for the time I am having. If I could live this last year again, of course I would like to skip the leukaemia, but many of the changes and discoveries I have made I value and would not wish to lose: a developing deep supportive faith in God, an even closer and more precious relationship with Ian, a very clear reminder of the love and support of my family, the continued loyalty of my old friends and the many new friends we have made along the way, and a close look at my life which is continuing to encourage me to examine myself and my priorities. Exciting stuff ~ long may it continue.

Robin's first day

A friend pushed the leaflet into my hand saying, "This might be of interest to you", and for a while I thought no more of it.

I was going somewhere else at the time, where you sat from 10 am to 3 pm with no one much who wanted to talk. There was a vicar who was chatty at lunch time and a few old girls you could make giggle if you tried hard enough. I said to my sister, who was looking after me at the time, 'I don't think I can stand much more of this', so one Tuesday we ambled along to Stockwell Street like Tweeddledum and Tweedledee. A Church Hall, though. I wasn't too sure about that. Churches aren't exactly my scene so it followed that Church Halls weren't either.

Grimly ~ and I've been told on a number of occasions that I looked worried and confused when I first came to the Centre ~ I pushed open the door on a big room full of books and chairs, in a sort of rough circle, and tables and …. people. People who came up, after they'd found us somewhere to sit, and talked to us. Yes, the other place had people in it and they were very kind and I don't want to knock what they were doing, but these people seemed somehow different. At first I couldn't really work out what it was but eventually the penny dropped. We were talking about this and that and how's your father and what the weather was like, and I thought to myself ~ shouldn't we be having serious discussions about our illnesses. Well, perhaps we did a bit from time to time, but most of the time it was idle everyday conversation.

And then, much later, somebody said, "Are you coming to have some lunch at the café?" The TopCafe, translated into Turkish as the Topkapi. That might have been the final thing that persuaded me.

Oh, and by the way, you can make the old girls giggle here if you try hard enough ~ not to mention the less old ones.

Ann responds ~

Robin handed this over and I read it as I made his coffee. Took his coffee into him as he was discussing fathers and being idle and I said, "I NEED TO KNOW, Robin, before I decide to either give you this coffee or throw it over you, if I'm one of the 'old girls' or the 'less old ones'. Fortunately for him he made a politically correct reply.

Margot reflects on her time at the Centre

*H*ow quickly and unexpectedly the Centre becomes a focus for welcomes, absences, and the everyday ups and downs of this world ~ a life-line for many during the 'downs' when there is always someone to share experiences, to 'feel' for you. There are healers giving generously of their gifts. There are others offering endless 'cuppas' and heaps of TLC.

For those feeling stronger there are valuable books and videos to explore, helpful dietary advice and counselling support. There are also notice boards loaded with social events and requests for help to man stalls, place collecting tins and bring in used Christmas and birthday cards for recycling.

I am reminded each Tuesday of the sadness and joy that I have been part of with the wonderful people here. Looking back I feel very grateful for the privilege of belonging to such a group. It has given me a purpose and proves that there is Life-After-Cancer.

Our Helpers

We advertise ourselves as a 'self-help' group,
and to a large extent this is what makes
our Centre work so well,
for it is through giving that we receive,
and through helping others
that we heal ourselves.

*W*hen we are desperately ill it is easy to imagine that we are useless. At the Centre we have found that there's nothing like feeling useful to revive a flagging self-esteem. New members soon find themselves helping in unexpected ways. Many are surprised that by listening to the experiences of others, they somehow feel better themselves.

There is a very thin line between those who come to our Centre for help and those who offer it. In a sense, all who come here are helped, and each one of us gives help in our turn. We used to talk about our 'volunteers', a term that has been associated with recruitment, selection and training ~ formalities that are perhaps not appropriate in our organisation ~ confusing too, for as one of our members once remarked, "I'm not sure whether I'm a volunteer or not".

As help is given in very many ways we relate more readily
to the word 'helper' than to 'volunteer'.

Helpers, we have found, 'emerge' when jobs are to be done. Or perhaps it's just that we make use of our collective skills. When Zena and Paula were with us, we offered reflexology and foot massage. Since they moved away, Margot has joined us, and hand massage has become popular. Amongst our members are those practising counselling and aromatherapy. Others, over the years, have kept our 'art group' alive. At one time Jean ran a special group for women who had breast cancer. Caroline closes our Wednesday sessions with relaxation and visualisation.

Healers are an important part of our support system.
We are very fortunate that they offer their help free of charge, requesting
instead a donation to the Centre's funds.

Suzanne, one of our healers, tells us ~

From a young age I was very sensitive to people's feelings and
emotions, which were frequently different from what they
outwardly conveyed. I found this confusing. When I began to train as a
healer I found that this sensitivity was a gift that I could use purposefully.
I first trained as a spiritual healer and intuitive counsellor, and later as a
Reiki practitioner. Reiki is a complementary therapy and as such can be
used in conjunction with any medication or treatment. Each person
experiences Reiki healing differently, in keeping with what they most
need, be it emotional, mental, spiritual or physical relief. Most often
people feel a deep sense of peace and relaxation, and it is often effective
in relieving tension and pain. Hopefully the healing energy that comes
through me will activate a person's self-healing abilities. After a long
illness, trauma, a course of medical treatment, or surgery, our energies can
become depleted. Healing is especially helpful in offering some restorative
help, like a tonic. I find this work deeply rewarding, and feel it is a
vocation for which I was intended. I regard it a great privilege to be asked
by someone to perform a healing.

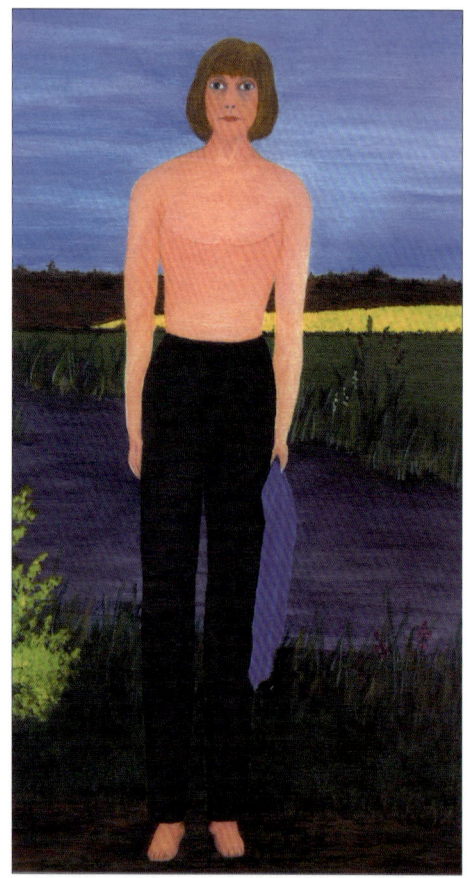

"Fenland Rising" (Self Portrait)

*Even after a double mastectomy, Fiona's self esteem remained
intact and she continued to see a beauty in her own body.*

The
Fighting Spirit

"I will seize fate by the throat;
it shall certainly not bend and crush me completely."

Beethoven

Recently Ann wrote:

A few years ago, sitting in my car at a busy traffic light in Central Cambridge, I saw a noble young man struggling with what looked like his first walk on two artificial legs. It was during the rush hour ~ lots of people must have seen him and agonised with him as he took every difficult heart-rending step. He was accompanied by a young woman *(perhaps a nurse)* who was allowing him to fight his way alone to unaided independence.

Each struggling step took him just a few crooked inches.

It seemed that he looked me in the eyes, and his expression said, 'Look at the hell I am going through! How can I bear it!'

I don't know how I didn't get out of my car to hug him and say, 'You are AMAZING. I admire you and the fact that you aren't despairingly in your bed, turning your face to the wall allowing life to zoom by'.

But the red light progressed to green ~ and another opportunity was lost.

S ince then I've learned all the appropriate words that go with fighting life-threatening illnesses. The most-used expression is, I suppose, 'fighting spirit', and evidence does suggest that those people with informed fighting spirit tend to do much better than those who are in denial.

Despite the nature of the illness ~ brain tumours, breast, uterine and cervical cancers, leukaemia, myeloma, lymphoma, oesophageal, prostate, bowel and bladder cancers ~ it seems that, fortunately, our Centre has a large share of fighting spirits. Certainly when most people come in for the first time they are overwhelmed by dread and fear. When they leave the Centre a couple of hours later, I believe ~ no, I know, that most of them ~ in fact all of them feel very much better and much more positive: they've linked in to the 'fighting spirit'

**Our Centre has developed over the years,
but that 'fighting spirit', which
was so much a part of the early days,
is still very much alive here.**

Rallying the Troops
by Supporting & Rousing

This was Ann's theme for a recent AGM Report. Here is what she had to say:

Supporting ~

I'm just going to say what I think we all know, but that if we are in a troop-rallying frame of mind it's good to remind ourselves of, that this Centre does its best to support those people who have cancer and those people who are carers of someone who has to face the cancer journey. I believe the support is particularly best given by people who have or have had cancer, backed up by those of us who haven't had to personally face the devastating blow of such a diagnosis. For example Gill, who was our first helper and who runs the Centre when I'm not here on a Tuesday, and Tricia who looks after everyone on Wednesdays when I am absent.

Perhaps it's helpful to remember Dulcie's comment a few weeks ago when she said, 'what is so special about this place is that it tries to provide for people's individual needs'. And I think well, we try but perhaps we won't always succeed, because we aren't perfect.

(As Ann often says, 'Nobody's perfect, but a team can be'.)

And then we come to:

Rousing ~

I'm not sure we need to rouse something that is obviously inherent at this Centre. But what we do in a gentle way is to awaken everyone's fighting spirit, rousing it into action, thus taking on the cancer and fighting it whilst at the same time *(and this is a big bonus)* we all make new friends and benefit from the contact we have with each other.

And the support and rousing comes in strong measure from people who are battling away against what they have to battle away at and yet they still find the time and inclination to put some, maybe a lot, of their energy into supporting other people, to show them what to do and how to do it.

And, yes, I do know that although a new person at our door may well have been asking themselves 'do I really need to go to this Centre?' before their first visit, they will leave with some joy in their hearts and a realisation that the visit was a good idea, that there is some hope emerging ~ and we should all be proud of that because to have that effect on someone, on many people, is incredibly inspiring.

What a team! Everyone plays a part. There isn't a single person at our Centre who doesn't contribute a sparkle to the success of this Cambridge Cancer Help Centre: our healers and counsellor ~ unpaid for what they do for us but certainly contributing in their different ways to our success, our librarian, who has set up our library in a proper manner, so that all our books are listed, labelled and cared for, and all those who collectively make tea, provide lifts, gather for lunches, dinners, social events, raise money, man stalls, make recycled cards, and try to put into action the most difficult skill ~ listening. What gems we have in this place. It is amazing. We all offer something different, because there are so many extraordinary ordinary people here to make the complete picture of a place that offers so much in such a loving way.

And another thing we have learned is that our informal way of going on is, for us, the best way of doing things, and that the person who has cancer is one of the best ambassadors for this Centre. Ours is the right way. And that Right Way didn't fall into our laps. We learned it through very difficult times. We devised it ourselves. Our Way doesn't appear in the text books on how to run a support group.

And the office team is the greatest of office partnerships. Tricia and I are able to share our strengths, admit our weaknesses to each other ~ not an easy thing to do for most of us perhaps but Tricia and I can do it easily and comfortably, and thus combine our strengths to work in the best way for the benefit of the Centre and the people who join us here. And our Trustees are, I can assure you, trustees of note, not just names that appear on the back of the newsletter. They all play strong parts in our rich tapestry, working away at all sorts of things that are part of the important background of the Centre ~ and with the good of the Centre at heart.

What a privilege it is to be a part of what goes on here. Can anyone wish for anything more rewarding and pleasurable, than to take everyone's side in their fight against cancer?

In the Snakatak café a little while ago about a dozen of us gathered for lunch, and because of the good-natured teasing a roar of laughter welled up from our little group. Such proof, you see, that our Centre isn't a dismal place but a place of hope and optimism and outstanding battling against the hardships our friends experience.

So my realisation is that in this very special place we do come together to offer support to the person who has cancer, and support to their carers, and we do hope to rouse them to fresh energy. And we do it our way, which is the right way for us.

All is well in this place.

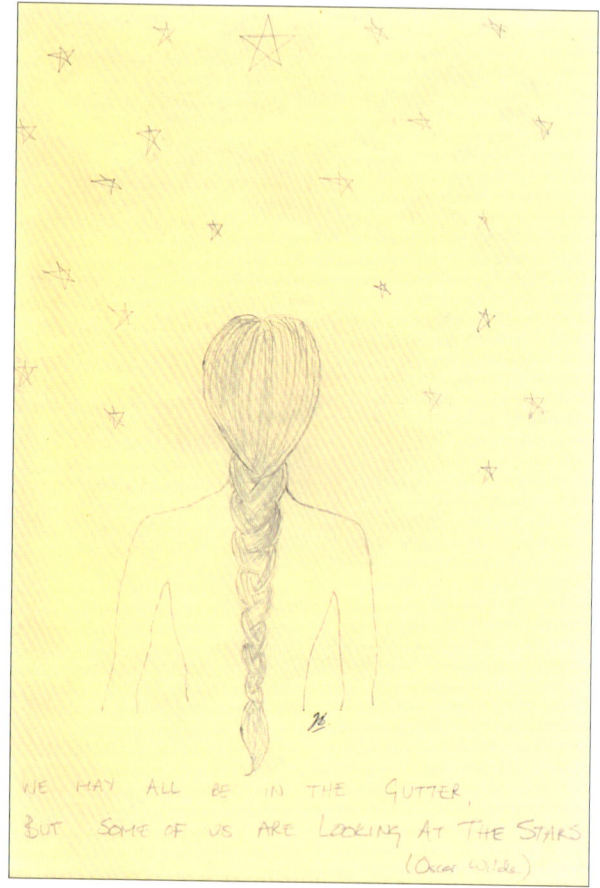

WE MAY ALL BE IN THE GUTTER,
BUT SOME OF US ARE LOOKING AT THE STARS
(Oscar Wilde)

"Looking at the Stars"

Fiona left this sketch abandoned on the table after a morning's art session. Fortunately Ann rescued it and felt very moved by it. It has been the inspiration for the title of this book and has been adapted by Daniel for the design of the front cover.

Some of Our Own Stars

Many of the stars here at our Centre continue to sparkle amongst us: others live on in our memories and through their writing ~ and through their partners who continue to find support within our group.

All remain an inspiration to the rest of us.

Judith's story ~
Shilstones Rocks Midsummer

Support, strength, and the will to overcome life's obstacles come in many different forms.

I was first admitted to Addenbrooke's hospital on New Year's Eve 1979. It was to be a routine operation to remove a malfunctioning thyroid, but it turned out not to be quite so straightforward. It was found to be a malignant tumour, and consequently I was bombarded with the full might of modern medicine. I had at that time three sons, aged one, three and seven years old, and also I had a pony. Officially she belonged to my children: in reality, she was mine. This equine was no sleek thoroughbred, but a typical Thelwell type. She did come with an impressive pedigree but over-indulgence and many babies had left her with a less than perfect figure. What she lacked in beauty she made up for in temperament and character. Her name was Shilstones Rocks Midsummer, Minnie for short, and she was due to foal again that coming Summer.

Strange as it may seem, my main concerns were for that pony, who was very special to me. I felt my children would be cared for, but who would take care of my friend?

On release from hospital and with no Cambridge Cancer Help Centre, to whom did I confide my fears? ~ to Minnie of course. Her big black eyes reflected love and concern, and together we helped each other. I was with her when she foaled and she was there for me when I needed comfort.

Life was good again. My treatments went according to plan and all seemed well. I can't begin to express my feelings when I found Minnie had a lump the size of a golf ball in her throat ~ in the region I imagined her thyroid to be. A visit from the vet and a stay at Madingley vet school confirmed she indeed had a thyroid tumour ~ benign or malignant they could not tell, but, as an operation was not a possibility, we had to adopt a 'wait and see' policy.

Fanciful as it may seem, I felt she had taken my tumour, but I was not prepared for her to die instead of me. She was as precious to me as my own life and I implored her to get better. The lump appeared to cause no restriction to her eating or breathing, even though it grew to the size of an apple. Then, miraculously, it stopped growing. Over the next two years it gradually shrank away, which none of the vets could explain. I felt we had both fought this disease and had both triumphed. She became my talisman. While she lived, I felt safe.

In July 1988, my husband and I took our three sons to the Ardèche region of France to canoe the white waters. We knew it would probably be the last holiday we would all spend together, as my eldest boy was approaching sixteen. It really was a very happy time, although I was terrified of the speed and the force of the waters. On our last evening, I became quite ill with stomach pains, which for me was very unusual. The next morning I awoke with my throat so constricted that swallowing was almost impossible. As we were leaving that day, it was decided we would get back home before seeking any treatment. During the journey home my husband enquired as to how I was feeling. To my astonishment, all symptoms had disappeared without my having realised. We arrived home in the middle of the night and collapsed straight into bed.

I was awoken early the next morning to be told Minnie had died. The vet had destroyed her, as she had developed grass sickness, for which there is no cure. Her symptoms were intestinal cramps and the inability to swallow!! She had been shot very near the time I realised all discomfort had left me.

I felt suddenly very alone and vulnerable. I didn't know what my future held without her. Our lives had become inextricably bound, and it seemed urgent to find another 'raison d'être', which came some time later in the shape of another horse, Willow ~ but that is another story.

This is my thanks and tribute to Minnie, who helped me through many dark days and whose memory I carry forever.

Much later Judith adds:

1 still have live cancer cells floating around in my system, yes. Does that concern me? Sometimes. I have had over twenty very good years since that first diagnosis. I have seen each of my three sons start school, progress to college and then jobs and manhood ~ something I thought I could only dream of.

My marriage has failed, but I have found new friends that are trustworthy, loyal and true. I have secured a job, which I love, and I have travelled to far-flung places. All of these experiences are more precious to me because I was brought face to face with the prospect of an early demise. On balance, my life has been more fulfilled because of my illness. It changed my thoughts, my aims and goals. The material things of this world were put into perspective, and for me the only reason for being is the relationships I forge with others.

I have very few regrets about the path my life has taken since being told that I had cancer. I cannot say that was true of my first thirty years, so maybe here lies the reason for my illness!

Life can be good after the 'Big C' but no one can tell how long that life will be. While it lasts, why not enjoy all the pleasures this life can offer, rather than live in the shadow of the universal truth that we will all pass from this life whether we have cancer or not.

Fiona's story ~ Living with cancer

I love my life. Each day makes me happy. Every day I try to live an expression of who I am. I call it 'living close to my heart', and it has been a wonderful revelation to me. And it doesn't take much to get me talking about it. Sometimes I see tears in people's eyes while I'm speaking. I hope that these aren't tears of pity, but are instead a sign that my words are touching people in a place deep down, a place not often visited in the rushing by of life.

Firstly the facts. I am thirty-six. My name is Fiona. When I was thirty-three I had been married for twelve years. I was living in a small village, working as head of a Speech Therapy Service in the NHS. If you'd asked me then how I liked my life, I'd have said it was pretty good. I loved my home and garden; I had wonderful friends; I liked my job; had no money worries; my marriage was OK; no health worries. If you'd pushed me a bit harder, I might have owned up to feeling the pressure of work more that I used to. As I gained promotion, so I gained more work, less time, more worries, more need to juggle ever-increasing demands and ever-decreasing resources. I'd have admitted that my marriage, though by no means terrible or fraught with rows or violence, had become more of a house-sharing than soul-sharing arrangement. I'd have acknowledged that whole weeks, even months, went by without my noticing; after all it's hard to keep count when days run together in a rushed cycle of home ~ work ~ home ~ cook ~ work ~ etc. If you'd really pushed me, and bought me a couple of drinks into the bargain, I might have told you that just occasionally a small voice from a place in my brain where my thoughts seldom went exploring, would whisper, 'Is this it then? Is this how life is going to be, and there's nothing I can do about it?' I was borderline unhappy ~ not sunk in misery, but like a tropical fish in a tidy tank, I sometimes had an inkling of something wider, some better, fuller, way of life, the consciousness of some vast ocean 'out there' where life was richer, but no idea of how to get there.

Then, just over a year ago, my husband and I separated. It was a shock at first, and I was angry and hurt. But after a short time I realised ~ or perhaps just admitted ~ that we'd stopped working as a couple long ago. I began to feel that this could be a new start, a chance to make some changes, changes that I'd been needing for a long time. I started to look for flats, contemplated changing my job and going part-time, returning to my painting, perhaps even selling some ..... I went to stay with my sister Joanna and we sat up late in the evening at her kitchen table, making plans.

A few weeks later, my world turned upside down. One Saturday night, I found a lump in my breast. I went to the emergency GP on the Sunday. The following week I had a biopsy. Two days later I saw the surgeon. It was cancer. A mastectomy was needed, and was planned for the following week. I felt fear like a snake uncurling and stretching in the pit of my stomach. I cried on Joanna's shoulder. I steeled myself for what was to come. I wrote lists of questions for the surgeon and got all the information about cancer that I could. I knew there was a chance it was curable. They would take some lymph nodes at the same time as the mastectomy to check if it had spread. I went into hospital for the operation, and hoped for the best.

After the operation I lay in bed frequently pushing the button that dispensed painkillers into my body. Princess Diana had just died. Her funeral was on every TV channel. The doctors came back with the news: over fifteen lymph nodes were affected. The cancer had spread. I came home to convalesce. After a few days I began to realise that my life had changed. Something had happened to me that meant I could never again take the future for granted. I needed to build a new way of living to fit this. My world had changed, so must I.

I started to read all sorts of books on dealing with cancer. Some of these talked about the connection between mind and body, what we think and how we feel. Thinking over all the times when rainy days had seemed great because I was happy, and sunny days terrible because I was sad, this made immediate sense to me. I started a notebook and wrote down things that inspired me. One of these, which I think came from Buddhist writings, was

"We are what we think.
All that we are arises with our thoughts.
With our thoughts we make our world."

I pondered this, and carried on reading more and more. I read about people who had overcome their circumstances. Some had recovered from cancer, some hadn't, but all had found ways to live happily and die with peace and serenity.

Meanwhile, I went to the Bristol Cancer Help Centre for a residential week. There I met others who were looking for a path through cancer. I was introduced to guided imagery and the power of my own mind. I received healing and felt the profound relaxation and peace it can bring. I ate healthy and delicious food and took advice on diet and nutritional supplements. Most of all, I was immersed in an atmosphere of love, care and peace. An atmosphere that said there are things you can do to help yourself. You do have power in this situation. You can choose not to be a victim. I continue to believe all these things to be profoundly true.

Once home again, I learned transcendental meditation and began to feel more in control, more able to start building a new life. Then came another blow. The cancer had spread to my other breast and another mastectomy was needed. Again, the fear that I'd begun to beat back awoke and stretched inside me. Another operation, but this time I used the meditation and imagery techniques I'd learned. The difference they made was startling! After my first surgery, I'd been in a lot of pain, and had such difficulty moving my arm that I'd been unable to drive for four weeks. This time, on coming round from the anaesthetic, I had to ask the nurse if the surgery had been done, because I felt no pain!

My time in hospital dragged because I felt better so much more quickly, and when I returned home, I was driving again within a week. The surgery had been the same each time. I am sure that it was my use of the complementary techniques that enhanced my recovery after the second operation.

I also used imagery in the subsequent radiotherapy and chemotherapy. While having radiotherapy I imagined the rays as cool mountain water washing away any unwanted cells and cooling and cleansing my body as they went. I had no burns from the radiotherapy. In chemo, I imagined the drugs as a golden liquid entering my body via the syringe and spreading throughout, destroying all impurities and bringing healing. Since that time, I have found that I have secondaries in my bones and abdomen, and have had to have further surgery once, plus two brief hospital stays. When I first found out about each of these, again the feeling of fear started, but each time it became weaker and weaker. I can say, despite the medical diagnosis, I continue to feel well in myself.

Over the last year I have learned so much, and have used other complementary techniques such as aromatherapy, ayurvedic techniques and herbs, reiki, kinesiology and nutritional support. I have received so much kindness and love, and my life has been changed by the fact that I know we are able to choose the life we lead, even in the most difficult of circumstances. I believe that we are here to learn to live as fully and completely as we can; to choose and build ways of living that express who we really are ~ allowing us to give out the love we all have inside us; to bring happiness to ourselves and those we care for, to free ourselves from fear, and to live 'close to our hearts'.

I can't claim that I am able to live like this all the time. There are times when I'm fearful or angry ~ times when I stop seeing the beautiful planet I live on and the wonderful people who care for me, and turn inwards ~ times when it can all seem too much. But I refuse to give up trying. And there are times, many of them, when I find myself very happy to be alive.

Here are a few ideas which have become touchstones for me in living with cancer. I often think about these in low times, and I really believe in them.

All of life is a risk. Although we usually go through life pretending otherwise, the truth is that life is a risky and unpredictable business. None of us knows what will happen tomorrow, never mind next month or next year. I am not saying that therefore it is wrong to plan for the future, only that it is wrong to live for it. Whether we have cancer or not, I believe we should focus more on the present than on anything else. In other words ......

Live for today. The past is over, and regrets about what's gone before waste energy without achieving anything. The future, good or bad, doesn't even exist yet. The only time we really have any control over is right now, so I want to live it as fully as I can. I try to do this by being more open than I used to be. I find myself noticing how beautiful is a tree, a flower, even the sky itself. I try to really listen to other people with different stories and points of view from my own, often finding that we've more in common than we might think. I've made some great new friends this way. Generally I try to focus on whatever I'm doing when I'm doing it, instead of only paying half attention, using the rest thinking about tomorrow or yesterday. This way I seem to get much more out of even small things like painting, gardening, going for a walk, or even cooking, which isn't my strong suit!

Get free from fear. I feel that fear is perhaps the biggest enemy we face living with cancer. But what is it we're really afraid of? For me, and I suspect for a lot of others, it's really fear of death. And yet we're all going to die some time. Healthy or ill, it's the one thing we can all be sure of! Before my diagnosis, I didn't think about it much. After my diagnosis, it turned into a major fear. I needed to work out how to deal with that fear. Firstly, I realised that death is part of our lives as humans on this earth ~ part of the cycle that we are all involved in, but don't discuss much *(especially in our Western society)*. Secondly, I realised that in fearing death, I'm really afraid of the unknown. And after all, no-one can tell us what death is like, or what it's all about. For me, this realisation has led me to investigate the spiritual side of my nature. I'm not a member of any religion, but I do believe in God ~ and in the human spirit. My readings in this area have opened up a whole new world of ideas for me, and though I can't claim to have the answers, I find that actually tackling spiritual ideas has helped me deal with that fear of dying, that I'm sure we all share.

Be true to myself. As time went by from my first diagnosis, I became aware that if I wanted to make my life as happy as it could be right now, I was going to have to deal with some personal problems and issues that I'd been carrying around for a long time. I talked about some of these to close friends, and gave them much thought. I also considered counselling as a way of getting to the bottom of some issues. Although I didn't end up pursuing that option, it's one that I think is invaluable for many people and I may try it in future if I feel I need to. One of my personal issues was that for most of my life I've looked after other people and put my own needs at the bottom of the list. Getting cancer made me see that this was not a good way to live, as I neglected myself and spent all my energy on others ~ *not* a recipe for success in living with cancer! So I started trying to put my own needs first ~ to say 'no' when I felt tired and somebody wanted me to do *x, y, or z* ~ and *not feel guilty* about it! To say 'I am important, and I'm still a good person' ~ to learn, as our American friends would put it, to 'love myself'. It sounds corny, I know, but it works!

I also had to tackle some problems in my relationship with my sister, that dated all the way back to our childhood. It wasn't easy, and we had some difficult conversations with tears all round, but we are now closer and understand each other better than ever before. I feel I've finally found out what 'being a sister' is all about, and it's wonderful!

Accept help. Finally, I've had to learn to accept help, and ask for it, without feeling guilty or a 'burden', or any of the other feelings that are common to those of us who are more used to being 'the helper' than 'the helped'.

Joining the Cambridge Cancer Help Centre was part of this for me, and being a member has helped me in so many ways that I'm glad I did! I've also learned to accept help from friends and family, and realised that doing so helps them as much as it helps me. Talking openly about the cancer to those around me, including my nieces and nephew *(15, 10 and 7)* has also helped. The children especially needed to understand what was going on. As I know, there's nothing so scary as the unknown. Understanding empowers us all!

My life didn't end with my diagnosis, though a certain way of living did ~ a way that no longer served my needs, and perhaps hadn't been serving them for some time. Cancer was the catalyst for me to take a long hard look at my life, and to see that I had a choice about how to live it. I've made a lot of changes, and am still making them, but I've no doubt that my life today is better now than it's been for years. I remember hearing someone on the radio express an idea that has become a fundamental belief for me ~

"The measure of life is not its length, but its content."

Ann reflects ~

Time after time we agonise with the women who lose their hair. We admire their wigs and then share their enthusiasm when the new hair, usually curly, appears. I remember being profoundly moved some time ago when two of them removed their wigs ~ on the spur of the moment, it seemed, whilst they were talking to the rest of us. What added to the emotion of the occasion was that it wasn't a case of all women together, sharing stories and experiences, but there were men there too, and I suppose that demonstrated the 'closeness' of the relationships we have at our Centre.

One of those women was Ingrid and here's her 'hair' story

Ingrid's story ~ Goodbye, Mrs Merton!

When I first heard I was going to lose all my hair due to the breast cancer treatment I was going to have, I wasn't too worried. I was more concerned with getting rid of the cancer and feeling well again. Before the hair loss took place I went with my daughter to the Wig Department at Addenbrooke's Hospital. We sorted through three or four different styles and decided on one which we thought suitable. With lots of giggles, we purchased the wig, along with a cleaner, and now I was set for the day when my hair would fall out ~ although at this stage I really didn't think it would.

Alas, after my first treatment, my hair started to fall out. But I thought I could hang on to it and decided not to comb, brush or wash it. The effect was yes, I kept my hair but it looked like a bird's nest, completely matted, dirty and smelly. When I went back to see the doctor at the hospital, after the second lot of treatment, he looked amazed and said, "You've still got your hair!" "Yes", I said, very pleased with myself. It was actually just lodged on to my head ~ almost as if it was a wig ~ only a very scruffy, tatty one looking and smelling like a dead cat.

Eventually my hair gave way to a windy day in the garden and it blew in great clumps over the fence into the neighbour's garden. I dashed to the nearest mirror. Oh, my goodness! I looked like some alien from outer space ~ and how cold my head felt. I actually felt sorry for bald-headed men ~ because of the coldness, I mean.

Next step ~ to try on my wig. It doesn't look like how I remembered it. I look like Mrs Merton. I try all ways to fluff it up and change the style, but it's still Mrs Merton. Oh dear! So I decide to buy a hat. First a woolly 'Benny' style for bed, as the pillow is freezing. Perhaps, I thought, some scarves would be good for the daytime and I managed to find a couple from the hippy years, tucked away in one of my drawers. They will do, I thought.

Everywhere I go I'm searching for hats and end up with about eight in all. Now that my hair has grown back, I cringe at the thought of ever wearing some of them. I think, my goodness, did I ever actually wear that awful hat?

On my brave days I actually went out in my 'Mrs Merton'. People, being kind, would say how lovely my hair looked, but I didn't believe them. The sweat would drip down my face from the heat of the wig and sometimes for sheer relief and devilment, when I was out, I would take it off, as if that was the natural thing to do and pretend nothing was amiss. People would look in awe at my shiny bald head and not say a word, and neither would I.

And then there were the remarks such as: "Have you lost your hair everywhere?" and I would hesitantly reply "E e e e e r - y e e e e s" and they would titter and giggle.

After eight months of trying to avoid mirrors and looking completely sexless, my hair started to grow ~ hip hip hooray! It was a slow process but at least it was growing.

I remember going out at one time with a friend who was at the same stage of hairlessness. We both had a Grade One haircut and people were staring at us, I suppose drawing their own conclusions. I remember going to buy some petrol and the cashier saying she admired my haircut but didn't think she was as brave as me, asking the hairdresser to style it so short. I didn't tell her the reason for my short hair. When it had grown a bit more, a man said to me that he liked my hair better now that it was longer. Again, I didn't let on.

Well, after one year, my hair is now back to its original state ~ thick, curly and wild looking, but I don't mind one bit. I will never moan about it again. Losing one's hair means that it's cheaper and easier to look after, with no haircuts, colours, shampoos and conditioners to pay for.

But I know how I prefer to be!

Some time later Ingrid continues her story ~

I have just, for the first time in my life, at the grand age of 50-something posed for some topless photographs. Unfortunately, I didn't get paid and I wonder why ~ maybe it's something to do with my age. If I was 30 years younger, I could have made a lot of money. 'Page 3' girl maybe? Wishful thinking, but these thoughts were running through my head as I posed, red-faced, with a lovely young photographer taking pictures. I expect you are wondering what the reason was for this procedure. All will be revealed later on ~ in more ways than one!

After two years, I have just finished the last stage of having breast reconstruction, after losing a breast to cancer three and a half years ago. While having an after-care check-up, I was asked by the doctor if I'd thought of having reconstruction. "Yes, PLEASE" was my eager reply. An appointment was made to see the plastic surgeon.

He explained two ways of doing the operation. One was by taking a muscle and a section of skin from my back, bringing it through to the front, then adding a saline implant. The other way was using a muscle and the fat *(plenty of that)* from my stomach, plus an implant and bringing that up to where my bust should be. I was given a book to read about both operations and was told to return in two weeks with my decision.

After reading the book, I decided on the first option with the muscle from my back, as this was where there was only a 1% failure rate against 20% with the stomach method, which I thought was quite high. *(It's possibly better now as this was some years ago.)*

Back I went with my decision and asked if I could see a photograph of the finished result but none were available. Luckily a patient in the next consulting room offered to show me her recent operation and it looked quite good. At that time there was a four to six month wait, but if a cancellation came up, I could have the operation earlier.

A phone call, after only three months' wait, told me there would be a bed for me that week. I didn't have much time to think about it, which was great. My only concern was that I was getting married in eight weeks' time, but they said I should be OK. Tony, my 'intended', thought he would be getting a better deal ~ an added bonus! I went into hospital on the Thursday and had the six-hour operation.

Because of the immense encouragement and support I have received from everybody at the Centre, I have managed to find sufficient strength as I've gone along. I always knew the Centre was an amazing place and now I've been reminded again why ~ it's the people who come to it. My fondest and sincerest thanks to you all!

p.s. The photographs of Ingrid were used for a medical text book.

Pat's story ~ Living with the enemy

Casting my mind back to that day in August 1989 when I found the lump and 'knew', as you do, that it was cancer, I went through the whole gamut of emotions, examined all the possible scenarios, decided it would be fatal, and accepted death as the inevitable. The doctor's confirmation that the lump was malignant brought me face to face with my two most immediate fears, telling my family, and facing an operation, having never had one. I was terrified by the thought of being put to sleep by anaesthetic. I was not going to have a lot of time to think about it, however, as an early date for an operation was offered by Torbay Hospital.

My family's initial and expected reaction was disbelief and distress, which then turned to practicalities, when my oldest daughter, a nurse, insisted on a second opinion in a London hospital. A hurriedly arranged consultation with a specialist at the Royal Marsden Hospital resulted in admission a few days later. So I quickly found myself on the cancer conveyor belt. A large lump was removed from my left breast by segmentectomy. Lymph drainage revealed a slight trace of cancer in one node. I was prescribed chemotherapy, radiotherapy and Tamoxifen, and, all the while, having to cope with the running of a 27-bed residential home for the elderly in Devon, whilst, at the same time, concealing my condition from most of the staff and all of the residents until the home was sold in February 1994 with all the attendant trauma.

Retirement to our small flat in London followed, and a few months later a move to a smallholding in Hertfordshire to satisfy my husband's need to be a farmer. Doing the books was to be my only involvement in this venture. Life became full again, you always fear it won't, when you give up a full-time and absorbing career. I could give my attention instead, to being a full-time grandmother to my youngest daughter's three sons, who lived nearby. Looking after a house and large garden, interests and hobbies all helped to fill the void.

I felt well. In fact, I have to say, I never had felt ill, never felt any pain at any stage. The chemotherapy was of the mild variety and the only side effect was the anti-sickness drug given to me after the first session. This had made me feel 'spaced out' and unreal to such an extent that when I was informed by the police that my Austin Metro had been stolen from outside our flat, pushed down a slipway into the Thames, and had been covered by at least one high tide, I simply smiled and said, "Oh, really".

So, I felt good, complacent even. The Marsden had 'fought' my cancer and won and I had unquestioningly accepted all the treatment my medical and oncology teams had decided on. They now kept an eye on me at the regular check-ups that followed in the succeeding years. All was well, or so I thought, until May 1997 when, as a result of having a bilateral breast reduction, more cancer was found in the left breast. For two weeks, I was able to enjoy my two beautifully reduced, perfectly shaped and well-matched boobs, before they whipped off the left one and replaced it with a nipple-less mound composed of an implant covered by muscle from my back. It had all happened so quickly, I had no time to think properly. "Are you absolutely sure about the histology results?" I questioned. "Oh, yes" I was told, "we don't make mistakes here". Was I being too hasty in having an immediate reconstruction? "Well, it's fairly normal now", they told me. "Don't worry, we will remove everything back to the chest wall before reconstruction."

In my confusion I agreed. I told myself it was lucky it had been found. But was it luck, or had I had a slight suspicion? Perhaps that was why I had persuaded my surgeon to do the reduction. Luck or what? I don't know. Then there was talk of possible secondaries. Scans, ultra-sounds and x-rays followed, then the wait, the fear again; the grim reaper loomed once more on the horizon.

All the mix of emotions, the tears, the soul-searching, then reprieve, nothing was found. God had been good. I had been given another chance and things were going to be different this time. I was going to fight for my continued health.

The reason for my getting cancer was something I had often reflected upon. There were no obvious clinical causes: I was not a smoker, had been a vegetarian for twenty five years, and because I had high cholesterol, I was on a very low fat diet. I had not, as far as I know, been abnormally exposed to chemicals or pollutants in the home or workplace. It had to be stress related. I had read that illness can strike when the immune system is low, and for a long time, I had been troubled by an incident that had occurred some months before the first appearance of the cancer. A chemical reaction had been triggered by the feelings of guilt and fear that I had experienced at the time and I had never properly dealt with it.

I sought out the psychiatric consultant at the Marsden and bared my soul. She reasoned and rationalised and tried to make me see that I was personalising my illness: it was fairly common for the patient to see themselves as the cause of their illness. Not totally convinced, I nevertheless felt better for off-loading my psychological burden.

Following the advice of another cancer patient, I booked myself into the Bristol Cancer Help Centre, whose holistic approach and combined mind, body and soul therapy has had much success in curing cancer. The benefits of my week there were immeasurable; the calming supportive atmosphere, the sharing of our experiences, grief and emotion, and the love that emanates from the healers and counsellors, the practical help from the doctors and the dietary advisors, the wonderful healthy and delicious meals, the emphasis on inner healing, the power of the mind, the benefits of relaxation, visualisation and meditation. After coming home, a changed woman and a convert, I adjusted my diet to a non-dairy, 95% organic one and commenced the recommended regime of vitamins and supplements, so I immediately felt I was doing a lot to help myself. Bristol also advised joining a support group. I checked out a few and finally found the Cambridge one, which felt like a home from home. Comfortable, friendly atmosphere, caring, knowledgeable helpers and healers, a varied mix of patients needing support, many of whom take part in fundraising and other events, and who in turn, become supporters to others.

It's a 45-minute drive from my home, but well worth the effort to travel there once a week, whenever possible. For two years running, a group of us has enjoyed a weekend away in Sheringham, which provides a very large dose of the best possible medicine ~ laughter!

Another of Bristol's recommendations was to find a holistic practitioner, and I have recently been able to achieve this as a patient at the Royal Homeopathic Hospital. I have also spent a week at Ickwell Bury in Bedfordshire, on a yoga course, and as a result, started going weekly for exercise sessions. As well as the obvious benefit, yoga teaches deep and correct breathing, ~ another must for cancer sufferers: cancer cells hate oxygen! A session of yoga aids relaxation and meditation. I work hard to achieve the inner stillness that aids the body's well-being.

Vigilance is needed in my fight against cancer. Having had one recurrence, I know I could have another. If there are any active cells in my body, I am ready to do battle with them. A recent scientific survey showed that a fighting spirit can reduce the chance of a recurrence by 80%. Doesn't that make it worth it?

Cancer was one of the main scourges of the 20th century and has not diminished as we enter the 21st. It would appear that there is not enough research into the causes, because there is more profit in the search for a cure. It may be that our health is being sacrificed to the financial interests of the chemical and nuclear industries, but we must not consider ourselves totally helpless as individuals, as we know that there is much we can do to help ourselves and, in seeking that help, we find ourselves and our lives can take a new and interesting turn, and a whole new world can open up when we join the cancer club.

This is the one nobody wants to join, but for some,
it can be a privilege to become a member.

A Whole New World

The life-enhancing qualities of the cancer experience
is a recurrent theme at our Centre

*David remembers that his wife Elizabeth used to say, "Cancer is the best
thing that ever happened to me!"*

David tells Elizabeth's story

C ancer made her stop and take stock of her life. She decided what she
wanted and how she was going to do it. Instead of, for the most part,
letting life just happen to her, she took charge. Only as far as her disease
and other circumstances permitted, naturally; but by comparison with what
went before, that is just what she did: she took charge of her life.

To begin with, Elizabeth gave up a very stressful job at the University
Press. She was good at it, certainly, but she could now do without it. She
did not give up work entirely. After a couple of months of blissful idleness
she went back to being a library assistant, something she had briefly done
as a teenager, and this she continued with as long as her disease *(and its
treatment)* would let her.

As a girl she had wanted to go to art college, but Father had put his foot
down; she had to qualify herself for 'a proper job', and so she went to
teacher training college instead. Until she had cancer, all she had time to

do was knitting, crochet and dressmaking, including making costumes for some of our historical dancing group. But now she went on a foundation course at the Open College of the Arts, and learned to paint in oils, acrylics and watercolour. Acrylics she did not take to, but some of my most treasured possessions today are oils and watercolours that she produced during those years. She also took up weaving and learned to do bead-embroidery. She probably did too many things to have time to find her own style in any of them. Time was not on her side, but her life was enormously enriched by this great burst of creativity, and so was that of those who knew her.

It was the same with her physical and spiritual health. She explored a great many ways of building up her immune system, eliminating stress, and achieving inner harmony and balance. She regarded diet as very important, gave up red meat and red wine and most dairy products, and tried a number of different dietary regimes. Elizabeth was not doctrinaire about such matters; she came to know what suited her and followed that. She learned to listen to her own body and did what it said. She had the same approach to complementary therapies ~ healing, acupuncture, aromatherapy, reflexology, relaxation, visualisation: she took what she needed, when she needed it. She saved up to go to the Bristol Cancer Help Centre. She went on a course in Scotland designed to reinforce the personality. She discovered transpersonal counselling and used auto-hypnosis. Here again, she took charge of her life and gave herself the best chance she could. As she said, "I have never felt so well. I am a very well woman who just happens to have cancer".

The one time that this did not work was during chemotherapy. Elizabeth was unlucky in reacting very badly to the treatment and felt awful for the best part of nine months. Furthermore, there was the basic contradiction that she was now voluntarily taking drugs that would weaken her healthy cells and degrade her immune system ~ the exact opposite of what she was in principle aiming to do. That was a bad time for her; she was often depressed and had a difficult time getting through it. It was such a wonderful relief when they stopped trying to treat the cancer and concentrated instead on giving her a decent quality of life for the time that remained.

Despite everything, despite acute discomfort in her arm from lymphoedema and from the cancer itself, despite growing shortness of breath as the cancer invaded her lung, and despite the ever more certain knowledge that time was running out, these times *(before and after chemotherapy)* were times of considerable happiness and fulfilment.

That is what Elizabeth had meant when she had said, 'cancer is the best thing that ever happened to me'. Cancer had given her the reason, and she had had the courage as well as the opportunity, to take charge of her life and make the most of what it could give her. She had five years from the time of her initial diagnosis, and, apart from 1992, in which the only good things were a summer holiday in Italy and Christmas in Dorset, they were some of the best and most rewarding years of her life.

Wendy's story ~
No longer an outpatient

*H*urrah. I am no longer an outpatient. About fifteen years ago, I had my third brush with cancer. My consultant told me I'd be lucky to live for five years. At first I refused the drastic surgery needed for my recovery, but gradually friends and family convinced me that if I wanted to see my young children grow up I should undertake whatever was necessary. So I did. I spent three months in hospital following very major surgery and complications and six months slowly recovering, putting one foot in front of the other, taking two steps forward and one step back. Bit by bit I improved, got stronger and gained weight, took up bits of my life again, and slowly came back into the world of the fit and healthy.

At first my check-ups were weekly then fortnightly, then monthly, then three monthly then six monthly and finally annually. I hated them. I would spend a week pacing nervously about the house, rehearsing what I would say if the consultant examined me and then asked me to come back into his office and bring my husband with me. I hated the smell of the place. I hated seeing nurses and doctors I knew from my previous visits, and remembering what they had said to me or how they had given me treatments. I hated seeing other patients with white, drawn faces, hearing their nervous forced gaiety, watching their loved ones looking equally anxious.

The day came for my annual check up. My previous consultant had retired. There was a new man. I did not know him. I felt I had to tell him my history, although he had the notes in front of him. He didn't know me. He didn't have the shared recollections I had with my previous consultant. I had built up an easy-going relationship with him. After all, he had known me literally inside out. We had spoken in the dark hours about my fears for myself, for my family, and my future. He had gently talked me through the prognosis. He had operated on me. He had celebrated my milestones as I recovered. What was the new man going to say? He told me to "push off". He said he thought that I had been well for enough years to be written off. I could come back at any time I wanted to if I had a problem. "Go away", he said, "and live the rest of your life"

Yahoo! Hip-hip Hooray! Yes! Sorted!

All those things. I'm no longer an outpatient ~
and I'm deliriously happy.

Ron's story ~ Thirteen years on

I was taken to Addenbrooke's Hospital on 25th January 1990. I kept losing my balance and falling over. When I used to go into the bathroom, I found I was walking backwards, but at that time, I did not realise that. I was told I had a dark object on the right side of my brain, but in front of that I was bleeding from a clot. I was not told that at first.

I saw the surgeon before the operation; a surgeon from Norfolk and Norwich Hospital came to assist. My operation took eight and a half hours. I was in the Intensive Care ward. When I regained consciousness, I saw two people near me. They had gowns and masks. I didn't know who they were. They held my hand; then one of them whispered, "Hello, Dad".

A few days later, I was put in a ward. When I could get up, the first thing I did was to go into the bathroom and stand at the basin to see if I walked backwards. No, I didn't. That was the start of my recovery!

I had to have a head mask made of a kind of plastic with slits in it where the radiotherapy rays had to go, and I was 'bolted down' before going into the scanner. Although it was for only ten minutes at a time, it seemed like hours, not being able to move.

However, after that, because I lived on my own, I stayed in the hospital to start chemotherapy. It didn't like me and I didn't like it. Because of the treatment, I had damage to the tissues of the central nervous system, which can never be repaired. Perhaps, one day, they will be able to.

My balance is not very good and I get a bit unbalanced but I can manage that. Also, my memory is poor, but once again, I can get by.

One of the most marvellous things in my life is my dear and lovely friends at the Cambridge Cancer Help Centre. I know I can trust them and rely on them. Thank you, all of you.

Adrian's story ~ Feel the force

The film 'Star Wars' and cancer are two subjects that are stored in opposing corners of my mind's virtual library. I would have previously been unlikely to think about these subjects on any given day, let alone simultaneously ~ the juxtaposition of frivolous light entertainment and soul crushing illness never having occurred. A few months ago though, my brain coughed and spluttered briefly into action to present me with a personal analogy that was, to me, striking.

The film 'Star Wars' features futuristic gladiators called Jedi knights. These people are born with what is called 'The Force' within them: it is in some ways their spirit. The Force is powerful and must be nurtured by the carrier, and it also takes years to learn to use it to its maximum potential. These knights are respected and they fight for what is just, but unfortunately some of those blessed with the Force veer to the 'Dark Side'. This is the same Force but it is evil and as strong as the good, and the unwary can easily be drawn into it.

Immediately after my diagnosis of testicular cancer I had no feelings of a Force. Later, after weeks of anxiety, I still had no Force. Months after, when the stress was making life a chore, and enjoyment of anything was difficult, my Force started to grow. Slowly but steadily I was sinking to what I now think of as the Dark Side. As my worry continued, the power of the Force grew as it fed off my turmoil, its gravity increasing and unavoidable.

My ever supportive wife suggested that the Cancer Help Centre at Cambridge could be worth contacting. That was a good call. From my first visit I felt a fresh hope, and on subsequent visits this feeling increased. My Force was still strong, but it was changing: it was starting to polarize to the positive side.

At just over two years following my diagnosis I feel that I control my Force. I can have fun, be constructive, think of the future and lead a life even better than 'normal'. Armed with the Force, obstacles are not so great. The present can be enjoyed.

I have sensed a Force in the inspiring helpers at the Centre, many of whom have had cancer themselves, and I hope that my Force may become as strong as theirs one day.

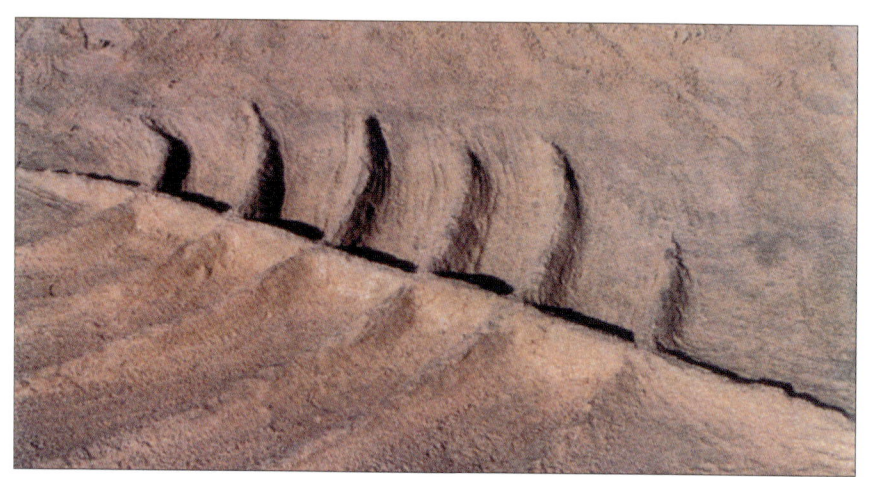

Anne

*comes to terms with her slow recovery
through her art.*

'Bones' or 'Inching my way along'

A t the end of August 2001 while on holiday in St. Ives, Cornwall, I made a sand sculpture on Porthminster Beach. It was my first piece of work in the landscape for several months as I had a breast cancer operation in April and radiotherapy in August. Before my diagnosis I had nine very stressful months in my life and was rushing around like a hare. But now I have become a tortoise ~ or maybe a baby turtle on a beach, inching my way along. The sculpture sums up to me how I feel I have convalesced ~ very slowly, but despite setbacks I am steadily inching my way forward! Thank you to everyone at the Cambridge Cancer Help Centre who has shown me such love and encouragement.

Patrick's story

*H*ere I am still, almost sixteen years after being warned that I might have only two years to live.

My problem was a tumour on my left hip joint, which though cured by radiotherapy, left a crumbled socket that was inoperable.

My anger at feeling cast on the rubbish tip led me to seek spiritual healing, and this helped greatly. I was put on a vegetarian diet with vitamin supplements, which I still follow. I felt well enough two years later to move from Oxford back to Cambridge.

Although I now have a severe limp and need walking sticks, I still manage all my housework and drive my car *(no automatic gears)*, but best of all is that my annual check-ups at Addenbrooke's Oncology Clinic show that my blood is testing normal.

Sometimes it is sad to hear from people who have had cancer, especially those who have had breast cancer, that they notice a lessening of touching and affection from those they hold dear.

Brenda *expresses this feeling in her poem*

Cuddles

All I want is a cuddle.
I had cuddles when I was a child.
I had cuddles when I was courting *(oh yes!)*
I had cuddles when I was married,
For twenty-five of those years *(oh yes!)*
Cuddles after that time were going;
Cuddles, now I am low ~ all gone.
Oh, for a cuddle.

Helen's story

R elationships at home were such that I could not share my worries and could not bear the thought of others worrying and making a fuss.

My mistake was finding this lump in August. Surgeons and consultants go on holiday in August, so there was a delay, but eventually an appointment came through. Still hoping this nightmare would go away, I went to the hospital by myself, telling my family that I was going for a 'check-up'.

When I was admitted to the ward, I thought it was the beginning of the end. During the day, deep depression set in and I ended up in the toilet, sobbing my heart out. I was found by a nurse and got a ticking off for being so upset. This made me angry. I had every right to be upset. I had carried this secret with me for three weeks ~ no wonder I was upset!

I was told I would go to theatre the next morning and that they quite expected my lump to be benign. However I was asked to sign a consent form, agreeing that if it was found to be malignant, my breast would be removed. Then the question came, 'What does your husband think?' When I replied that he did not know, the staff were not happy with me.

I remember waking up after the operation and the doctor coming round and saying, "I'm sorry". That day and night were miserable. I felt depressed and was unable to move because I was so sore. I had hit rock bottom. I have to say that the staff were excellent ~ but then, I don't think you come across bad medical staff.

I didn't enjoy the visitors who came and sobbed all over me. Some of them I hadn't seen for ages: neither have I seen them since. It felt like being a corpse in a coffin at your own funeral and they were coming to say 'goodbye'.

My daughter had a fear of hospitals and did not visit, but my son and his friend came to take me home. I felt very pathetic in my grey suit, which did not fit because I had lost weight. Also I was sore and didn't want the clothes to touch me.

It was good to get home and I remember thinking 'perhaps everything will be all right now ~ I won't have to struggle to keep up with all the housework and perhaps husband will take me out more and we can go on holiday'. What a laugh! Everything was just the same as it had always been. The cat still had worms, the fluorescent light bulb still did not work and the garden was a mess. I propped myself up on the settee with cushions and, of course, husband had to dash off to feed the horses. Sometime during the next few weeks, I remember asking for a cup of tea, and someone, perhaps one of the children, saying, "What's wrong with you ~ you've got arms and legs, haven't you?"

Home life got no better and the children dashed in and out for meals and clean clothes. Bank Holidays, Easter and Christmas were always a nightmare. I'd look forward to them, go over the top with decorations, cooking and presents, and it always fell flat with no support from the family. I realised I was beginning to feel very old and I did not want to end up as a pensioner sitting by the fire with no company and no interests.

I started going to Country music evenings with a friend who'd lost her husband. We enjoyed our outings and travelled the country, meeting many lovely people. The only problem was coming home. No one ever said, 'did you have a good time?'

The instructor at the *(line dancing)* class was alone and so was I. Out of that friendship came a permanent dancing partner. I realised that I was leading a double life and, more and more, there seemed no reason to go home. Eventually I moved into rented accommodation. I walked away from the family home taking some ornaments, two knives, forks and spoons, two cups and saucers and plates, a sewing machine, Grandad's armchair and a single bed. Looking back from a distance of twenty years I don't know how I did it. I must have received hidden strength from somewhere to go through this chapter of my life. I firmly believe that if I had not had cancer, I would not have been so positive about turning my life around.

And it was a good move. I was able to share my problems with my dancing partner and best friend. We are now completely sharing our lives and are lucky that our extended families are supportive.

There was light at the end of a very dark tunnel after all.

Living to be 104 ~ by another Brenda

*I*t is wonderful to be welcomed into the family of the Cambridge Cancer Help Centre. One of the very positive things is being able to share your ups and downs and laugh at life's tricks and treats.

We were talking about dreams while sharing a meal at the 'Caf'. I don't dream often but the ones I remember are important. One month before my breast cancer was diagnosed I dreamed I was sailing towards a beautiful river mouth over a smooth blue sea. I looked forward to exploring the hills and woods I could see from the glass room in the bow. To my amazement the ship ran up the beach and stopped. "I will die, this glass won't hold the list of the ship, I'll be crushed", I thought. But everything just went still.

And that is what happened in my life. My life as a busy GP stopped and I went through six months of treatment and recovery. I came out of these knowing I had beaten it and life would go on. But other things had also changed. The NHS was ailing ~ getting the right treatment for patients was becoming more difficult. Practising holistic medicine became increasingly more stressful. Society seemed to be breaking and hurting people more by setting money values above valuing each person for who she/he is. Those wounds are hard to heal.

I became very tired. Three years after my breast cancer I was diagnosed with small B mantle cell lymphoma. This felt much more serious. I retired as a 'burned out' GP and set about getting better.

I contacted the Bristol Cancer Help Centre *(this brought me to the Cambridge group),* found out about juicing diet, vitamins, keeping active, praying, meditating and visualisation. So I juiced and prayed and rested. I started looking after myself and finding joy in life again. I visualised my cancer cells as poor and tired, easily destroyed by my mighty T killer cells. But I didn't feel right. My body had been my most trusted, faithful *(and 'abused')* buddy all my life. Why was it turning against me now? I read the books of Le Shan and others. Yes, there definitely had been times I was tired of life ~ and that would not have helped.

Then I realised I had never really looked after myself properly, never stood up for 'me'. Work, family, pets, the house and garden and … always came before what I might need for me. My little lymphoma cells were hanging on trying to defend me, making antibodies: maybe even my T cells were worn out too. I should be grateful to them, because they tried to fight for me when I couldn't be bothered. Because I allowed myself to retire, because I had a second cancer, I was ~ am ~ happily alive now. Struggling on with work might well have killed me otherwise, and so I loved them and said thank you.

I have got the message now. From now on I will take care of myself; say no if I don't want, or would have to struggle, to do something; allow myself to do things I really like; to eat the right things and enjoy all the treats ~ and have the naughty ones too. Now those cells would be at rest and follow their natural pattern and die in peace, with my blessing and gratitude.

I have given that little thought since. I garden, enjoy my children, family, friends and pets. I have had some great holidays. At Christmas and New Year we celebrated how wonderful life is.

I woke early on the first of January, dreaming I had met my 'health visitor' unexpectedly. In her I recognised features of several nurses and health visitors who had helped me over the years. She was thrilled and surprised to see me. I felt surprised because I was feeling well. "But I was there with your diagnosis in the hospital", she said. "I saw your papers. Your cancer is all over you. There's no treatment or cure. They sent you away to live what life there was left. I thought I would never see you again." I tried to reassure her and told her I was better, really better. "In fact", I said, "I am well". I have never had such a deep 'gut' feeling about anything.

I woke up. What a strange and emotional dream. Had I been fooling myself that I could be better and live life to the full? It played on my mind for several hours. Then it struck me. She had been speaking the truth. She had not said anything I did not know. If that was true, then what I said was also true. I am better. That felt so right. I slowly started to glow and felt very happy. That feeling has not really left me since. Clinically it can never be proven. The only proof is in the 'Living to be 104 years old' and in beating all the odds.

And that is what I am going to do.

Carolyn's story

If you can't f***ing do it, then I will f***ing do it myself

*B*ack in September 1996, having just returned from Ecuador to my home village in the North of Scotland, I started having almighty headaches. I went to the doctor and she asked me to come back in two weeks if things didn't get any better. I said, "I don't think I can last two hours", but it didn't make her concerned. I travelled to Aberdeen to meet my sister, and after being sick one night in a taxi, we decided to go to A & E the next day. However, the receptionist was so snotty about me being there for just a headache that we left and went to my sister's doctor instead. He thought I might have a migraine and gave a prescription for this. It did help a little bit.

I returned home where I was living alone and I started having flashing colours across my eyes as well as the headaches. I went to see my doctors again and again but they just dismissed me. Eventually one doctor decided to send me up to the hospital for a CAT scan. At the hospital they did all sorts of tests on me. They tested my reflexes, getting me to follow a light with one then the other eye closed, and I 'passed' all of them, so instead of getting a scan I was sent home.

As time went on my headaches became more painful and frequent. On Christmas Day I couldn't go with my family to my cousin's for dinner but later on, I did go. I was sick yet again even on the small amount of food I ate. On Christmas Day we always have a game of 'Trivial Pursuit' and this question came for my team,'Who wrote Pride and Prejudice?'. I couldn't seem to retrieve the answer, but I knew that it was one of my favourite authors. I knew then that something was very wrong with me. On Boxing Day I just couldn't get out of bed so I asked my father to call the doctor. He was being put off on the telephone because he suggested I should be seen the next day, but my sister just grabbed the telephone and said, "we want a doctor, and we want him straight away". God bless her. The doctor arrived and I was sent into the hospital immediately for my scan.

It turned out that I had a large brain tumour, and luckily there was a surgeon who would operate on Hogmanay *(31st December)*. I think I went into blocking the whole thing out and just did what my family and the doctors told me to do. I had my operation and to my family's great joy I came out of it okay. I must admit I went a bit mad after the operation, which wasn't surprising after someone had just been working on my brain.

I was given radiotherapy and chemotherapy and then at the end of April 1997 I had a fit, which I don't remember, but my dad most certainly does. I awoke in hospital the next day and couldn't talk or walk, as I had right-sided paralysis. Immediately the oncologist told me that there was nothing more they could do for me. My radiotherapy and my chemotherapy hadn't worked. I think up to that point I had just put my life in the hands of the doctors.

But now I just thought "if *you* can't f***ing do it then *I* will f***ing do it myself". I think that was the point when I decided to live.

When I was released I made a point of thinking everything through because it was *my* body. I was at last given carbamazepine tablets and went on with a will to survive.

I was very slow and had to walk with someone helping me. I couldn't talk but boy, oh boy, I could swear. Apparently swearing takes a totally different path through your brain. And I could sing. Singing was something I had never done because I thought I was rubbish at it, but desperate needs ~ so I sang.

I was surrounded by relatives in the village that I had always called home, and each and everyone of them did everything they could to help me. They did this by taking me shopping and just being there for my family and me. My sister suggested that I go to a healer but I didn't want to go. She said I could just go four times and if it did no good then I needn't go back. The first time I met Elaine, my healer, I just looked at her cynically. But after the healing I did feel, remarkably, different. My cheeks were glowing and my eyes were sparkling. So, I went every week, and began to look at healing in a different light. I thought, right, if I get well, I will become a healer and pass on this marvellous gift. Every day I was managing to say one or two words and it was really marvellous because I am naturally a person who likes to talk a lot.

In the Summer my dad said he would let his sailing boat remain in the harbour for this year. I said "no" and that we should go sailing *(in not so many words)*. I had to be winched aboard the yacht. I'm glad that my father decided to go: everyone said that he was doing a stupid thing. My father said that if it was good enough for Francis Chichester *(who was diagnosed terminally ill with cancer and survived it by going on a voyage)* then it was good enough for him and me. In the end we set off from the village on the far north-east of Scotland with my dad and my uncle Billy and travelled about thirty miles a day down the coast of Scotland, then England and then over to Calais. Here we took out the mast and went motoring through the French canals, eventually getting to Paris, where we stayed for six weeks. I must say that I was never frightened of the sailing but I was absolutely terrified by the ladders going up harbour walls. But ~ I was getting some of my strength back.

When we returned home I decided that I couldn't stay in our village any more because I was too reliant on other people. Now I was getting better, I thought, I should move to another place, and my best friend who lived in

Cambridge suggested I should move down to stay with her. It was a big step but I did it. It meant I could use buses and my darling tricycle 'Buttercup' to get around as I was without a driving licence because I had experienced fits. The first thing I did was to find healers at the Cambridge Cancer Help Centre and at the Andreasen Centre, and I also attended the hospice's day care centre.

I learned how to become a healer and a counsellor myself. Now I have been in Cambridge three and a half years and I live in a Women's Housing Co-operative.

Earlier on this year I was given a driving assessment. It was really quite hard with about thirty tests given by an occupational therapist and then a drive with a driving instructor. And at the end of the day I PASSED! I have only been given my licence back for a year because of the type of tumour I have, but I will take another test at the start of next year.

I can now talk and walk perfectly but it took a lot of work. I still see the oncologist regularly and have been told my tumour is inactive at the moment. I put myself on an equal footing with everybody around me. It is my body and I must be consulted on everything. I am indebted to so many people who helped me get through this: my father, sister and brothers, all my relatives and friends, my doctors, the people in the hospices both in Inverness and Cambridge, Elaine and Penny who were my healers, and the healers I have at the moment, the people in the Cambridge Cancer Help Centre and the Andreason Centre and last, but not least, God, who delivered to me this little miracle that is still going on.

Carolyn is one of the healers at our Centre ~ one of several who give their time freely. She is a gentle, lovely person who is very moderate in her language!

A Carer's View ~ from Margot

It happened out of the blue ~ for the first time in our lives we had found undying love. What a joy it was ~ filled with adventure and challenges!

We had been married for three years when Dan's health deteriorated dramatically after he challenged his body by taking up long-distance cycling again, completing the London to Cambridge run. His sights were set on "London to Paris ~ Rome".

Investigations finally culminated on Christmas Eve, our third wedding anniversary, when we arrived at Papworth hoping for surgery. Alas, the screens showed liver involvement and I JUST KNEW. But Dan said, "Well, if I have cancer we shall challenge it." A clear message to everyone ~ "IT IS ONLY A WORD, NOT A DEATH SENTENCE".

During the following six months we explored many complementary therapies, including psychic healing, meditation and visualisation. Dan continued to contemplate Buddhism and other world religions and philosophical systems and to extend the spiritual side of his nature. But within horoscopes and the tarot he found predictions of his approaching death.

We benefited from a visit to the Bristol Centre, although it did have one unexpected outcome: after putting some rejected 'Bristol diet' out onto our bird table, we 'lost' the flock of starlings which used to eat there. The flock left abruptly and didn't return! A happier outcome was that we were introduced to the Cambridge Cancer Help Centre.

We nurtured, rested, examined our Inner Child, made peace with so many people.

I had support from a skilled counsellor and my sessions with her took place away from the house. Dan was unable to be left alone so I asked his daughter to come and sit with him while I was away. A major spin-off from this was that Sarah was able to renew and rebuild the relationship with her father that had been split asunder by a religious sect years before, which had isolated Dan from his family. All four of my step-children came for Father's Day a month before their father died. It meant a great deal to them and to Dan.

Shortly before his death Dan awoke one night and asked me to lay him out when the time came! ~ took a bit of time to think that out after forty years! However his oldest son and I arranged it. We compromised by mutual consent and with the help of the Natural Death Handbook (ISBN 071267111-0).

The 'Celebration of Dan's life' was conducted by our Buddhist friend, and included many more of varied faiths ~ a wonderful occasion in which we all participated. Cremation was followed by his ashes being placed in Wandlebury around a huge beech tree where we used to go for meditation and visualisation ~ and which is now grazed by sheep.

Helping relatives and friends and loved ones at the end is an important part of life. Knowing that it is their last journey may cause some to appear withdrawn. But they need peace and our presence along with expressions of love. And, at the end, permission to 'let go'.

I am a different type of carer now, committed to the weekly role of massaging hands at the Centre. This is a therapy for both patients and carers: it helps us all. There are many ways we can help smooth the lives of others, and so much joy in being involved in the process.

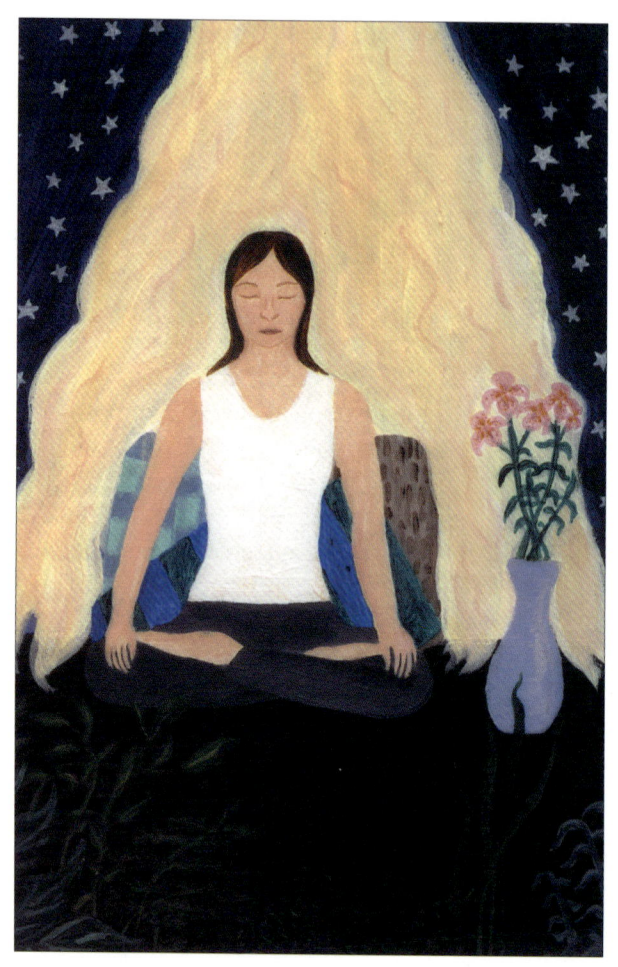

"Meditation"

Helping Ourselves

"The body has within itself the power to heal."

Hippocrates 500 BC

"Perhaps the most important thing about our Centre is that it instils in us the idea that we can help ourselves. Most of the ways we find to help ourselves are simple, but some require effort. This self-help gives us control of our lives again."

Marilyn

---

*I*an once remarked that at the Centre he had noticed that we try to listen to everyone's ideas and philosophies and treat them all with respect.

We believe that it is important for each of us to find and follow what makes our own heart sing ~ and a lot of 'singing' goes on at our Centre.

We do try to listen to everyone and take account of their views. We are careful not to push anyone in a direction that they feel uncomfortable with. For some people, the Centre provides their first taste of a spiritual approach to life. Others, coming to the Centre for the first time, are very sceptical about complementary therapies, which we encourage as a way of demonstrating that even at the blackest times we do have some control over our lives.

We stress that 'complementary' does not mean 'alternative'. We recognise the wonderful work being done by our medical teams, and although we do not give medical advice ourselves, we can put people in touch with those who are able to offer help.

To us it makes sense to use *all* the means at our disposal

Some years ago Keith recalled ~

When I was loading my things into the boot of a taxi which was about to take me to Addenbrooke's for my biopsy, I managed to cut my thumb on the inside of the boot lid. I thought no more about it until the end of the week's stay, when I noticed that my thumb had healed over completely. I suddenly thought, 'Well, I healed my thumb. No amount of medical treatment could have brought about that healing process. So if I can heal my thumb, there's no reason why I shouldn't be able to heal any part of my body that's gone a bit wrong.'

At that moment I realised that I should help my body to help itself as much as possible. It was an important step, realising that, together with the best support the hospital and others could offer me, there was no reason why Clarissa and I couldn't defy the so-called inevitability of the steady decline. I was completely flabbergasted at a conference recently in which a health professional used a chart which consisted of a dead straight line, from top left to bottom right, to describe a decline in health as time went on that was labelled the 'Cancer Journey', 'dead' being the operative word. But we were determined to prove from the outset that there are plenty of routes off that line and upward into health.

At the diagnosis day meeting, we bombarded the surgeon with questions, Clarissa and myself taking it in turns rather in the same way I like to believe 'tag-wrestlers' operate. When one of us was taking stock, the other would keep up the onslaught.

When it was one of my turns, I quoted the 'Heisenberg Uncertainty Principle' at him. In 1932, the German physicist Heisenberg was awarded the Nobel Prize for coming up with the idea *(to cut a long story very short)* that on any given curve on a graph, there is the possibility that one of the points that belongs to the curve is actually way off the edge of the paper. To put it into a more local context, I can do no better than quote a piece of graffiti asking, in relation to the college furthest from the centre of Cambridge: 'OK, Heisenberg, so where is Girton?' I explained to him that I had every intention of being a point well off the end of the 'mortality curve' I was supposed to be on.

Above all, I was *(and I am)* convinced that only a tiny part of my body had gone wrong, that it was my body so, just like my thumb, there was every chance that my body could sort itself out ~ with a little help from my orthodox and complementary friends ~ and that, provided I could look after my body as well as possible, there was no reason why I could not be the exception that proves the rule.

*B*eing diagnosed with cancer suddenly brings life into very sharp focus, and for many, is a wake-up call that sets them on a new path of self discovery. Few could have been more dedicated and meticulous in his search for answers than Keith. Eighteen months after his initial diagnosis, and having read over 70 cancer-related books, he produced his own list of positive strategies and therapies which he'd explored with his partner Clarissa, to complement his orthodox treatment: it makes impressive reading.

Here is *Keith's* list which originally appeared in one of our newsletters under the heading

'Complementary my dear Watson? ~ Highlights from a BTF member's diary'~
(BTF ~ Brain Tumour Foundation)

With help from the Oncology Department we contacted the Cambridge Cancer Help Centre, who in turn let us have nutrition and vitamin advice from the Bristol Cancer Help Centre.

We attended 'The Question of Hope' conference organised by Bristol and met the inspirational Gawlers and Candace Pert, amongst others.

I started a three-week exercise regime at a local gym, mainly on rowing machines.

Encouragement:
We received a consistently high level of support and encouragement for our tactics from our excellent quintet of consultants and duet of GPs.

I received further encouragement from ~
learning transcendental meditation
revisiting my spiritual roots by attending my local Methodist Church
starting a series of fact-finding longhand letters, generating 282 categories
of information to date!
reading Jenny Cole's pace-setting 'Journeys (with a Cancer)', which shows
what can be achieved with a determined attitude
receiving distance healing
joining series of workshops by Dr. Christine Page, on intuition, vibrational
medicine, and getting the most out of life!
meeting a crystal healer at Mind-Body exhibition, and starting a collection
of crystals.

Research:
I contacted 'New Approaches to Cancer' and received, apart from much other encouragement, a copy of *Consider This ...*, presenting comparative overviews of complementary therapies.

I also ~

got in touch with research organisations, receiving advice, abstracts and
papers
tapped into Bristol's newly-launched Mind-Body database
monitored relevant media items
joined the National Cancer Alliance, linking all interested parties
contacted Brain Tumour Foundation (BTF) and became a 'Brain Buddy'
kept a daily journal.

Normalisation:
As part of my pioneering 'normalisation' technique, in which I get to act like anybody
without a tumour, I continue to enjoy holidays, walking and taking photos in the
countryside, concerts, shows and funny films and cooking vegetarian meals.
I also ~

use a variety of music and other tapes in 'relaxation' sessions
maintain 'visualisation' exercises, in which I see my tumour as a poor,
confused little frog that has accidentally hopped into my head, and
which will hop out again soon!
have reached a personal best by rowing 2km in 8min. 23sec. in an
'Alternative Olympics' at the gym

And I feel privileged to have worked with a leading yogi at a Yoga for Health Foundation
Festival.

Vibrational:
I have spent an idyllic weekend African drumming in darkest .... Somerset.
I have also ~

had my voice analysed and received tailor-made Signature Sounds tapes
with specific healing frequencies
attended sessions in Bedfordshire with a colour therapist who uses crystals
and other therapies
have had my aura revealingly photographed before and after Reiki healing,
and learned Reiki 1st degree myself ~ all in Scotland!
visited Harry Oldfield and had illuminating PIP scans taken, and received
electrocrystal therapy
participated in a Matthew Manning healing circle and subsequent
one-to-one sessions.

Keith goes on to say ~

*T*he above mix of treatments *(revolving around vibrational therapies using sound and colour, crystals, electrocrystals and healing)* has been arrived at after much research. Although others will prefer different approaches, this works for me!

My application to retire on ill-health grounds was approved in record time, ending fifteen years in State music education, including two as an advisory teacher. I'm now aiming for fifteen years in cancer education, helping others to find out more about what they can do when confronted with adverse diagnoses.

The Brain Tumour Foundation knows that education about cancer issues is vital, and if I could help fellow patients track down advice at those times when they need it most, then perhaps even more good might come from that initial diagnosis of eighteen months ago.

*T*he irrepressible Keith never wavered in his determination to overcome his cancer, helping others as well as himself along the way. He continued, to the end, to follow what made his heart sing. Those of us who took part in an evening of drumming will remember with pleasure how he led us through a variety of rhythms, encouraging us to produce a creditable performance at the end of the evening.

This is how Keith described the occasion ~

One of my great interests as a secondary school music teacher was ethnic music of all kinds, but in particular those varieties from Africa. Indeed, as part of the therapies which we enjoyed in the aftermath of my diagnosis, my partner and I had worked with an expert in the field on two 'African drumming' weekends. So I knew exactly what I wanted to do as my 'party piece'.

My plan was to let all those who could attend enjoy the entrancing effects of the repeating rhythms and musical 'conversations' found in much African music. Upon arrival, I suppose some of the 'audience' may have been a little alarmed to find bongos, djembes, cabashas, dholaks, agogos and claves placed in front of their own chairs! But having spent fifteen years encouraging *(admittedly younger)* performers to enjoy the thrill of live music-making, I wasn't going to miss the chance of involving everyone in playing those instruments. I'm really grateful to them all for making it such an enjoyable experience for me!

In fact I was amazed at the sensitive and musical contribution of everyone to the improvised pieces of music we performed together. For instance, not once did any sounds continue after the signals to end the pieces, which shows acute listening and a high degree of concentration. More than that, there was a genuine enthusiasm to join in the playing by using appropriate and sympathetic styles of performance. Despite the unfamiliar nature of the music, I was delighted with the atmosphere we created. For me, it seemed that for an hour or so, we had transported ourselves from our busy lives, to a calm, unhurried place far away. This brought to my mind an expression I had recently heard:

'We have watches and clocks, but the Africans have time'.

The quality of authentic music-making that we successfully achieved was made possible by the generosity and kind support of the people at the local music shop, who lent us twenty-one instruments retailing at £1200 for absolutely nothing ~ a staggering sign of their support for our cause!

Fiona's way of dealing with bad news ~

*H*ow do we deal with those times in the 'cancer journey' when tests or scans give bad news, instead of the hoped-for good news?

Like many of us, this is something I have experienced several times. Firstly, a scan showed that the breast cancer, following my two mastectomies, had spread to my abdomen. Then further tests showed some secondaries in bones and lungs. Later following a period of 'partial remission' when these secondaries seemed to be shrinking, a routine scan showed they had started to grow and multiply again. Finally, and most recently, a biopsy to see if I might be suitable for a very promising new drug treatment came back negative, and therefore I would need to go on to a new chemotherapy regime.

I know that many others in our group have had similar setbacks to these, and I guess, like me, you may have found this kind of news hard to take. But what can we do to help ourselves over the initial shock and back into getting on with the rest of our lives? I have been thinking about the things that have helped me and thought I'd share some of these ideas with you.

Thinking through time. Each time I have had news of this kind, my first reaction has been a kind of mini-shock; a period when I've felt numb. I think this must be a way of allowing myself time to take in the news that I've been given and to think about what it might mean in the longer term. I think it's important at this time to discuss fully with the doctor what the results mean and what treatment may be on offer. If you're too shocked to talk at the time, make another appointment to see him/her another day, or talk it over with your Macmillan nurse or any other professional who is closely involved. As ever, understanding reduces fear.

Consider how the news impacts on every day life. When I got the news just after Christmas that my secondaries were growing again, I was very low at first. But then I started to think about how much difference knowing this made to my everyday life. Fortunately, I had experienced only a small increase in pain and this was well controlled by my drugs. I could still paint, garden, drive, visit friends and family, shop; in short, do everything I was doing before I got the news! So really, my daily life was as good as it had been before and this thought really helped.

You can choose how you think. Of course, my scan results mean my prognosis is somewhat worse than it had been. But, as I've said before, and really do believe, spending today worrying about tomorrow is a waste of the life I have. Whatever my prognosis, the future remains as unpredictable as ever. The only time I have any control over is now. I want to make the best I can of each day as I live it. I am convinced that thinking like this helps me to get the most out of life. The way we think about ourselves and our lives directly affects the way we feel and I have to admit that, most of the time, I feel very happy!

Asking for help and support. However, despite usually having a very positive view of my life, the times immediately after getting bad news have seen me feeling pretty low on several occasions. At these times, I have needed the support of another person and, for me, that has been a very dear friend, who lives fairly close to me. Just being able to phone her up or have her come round has been a huge help. We haven't always had an especially detailed conversation, but just having a shoulder to cry on or someone to give you a hug goes a long way. We must never be afraid to ask for this kind of help. Many people are only too happy to give it ~ they're just waiting for us to give them the sign.

Giving help and support. If there is one thing that is only too true in life, it's that there are often other people with worries and problems even more pressing than ours. When a friend of mine, who was going through some very hard times, rang up for a chat, I found that being able to offer her some support helped me too! Whatever our situation, we can always offer love and support to others.

*F*iona also found that certain poems helped her. Here is one she often quoted: it never failed to raise a smile.

> *"Yesterday is history*
> *Tomorrow is a mystery*
> *But today is a gift ~*
> *Which is why we call it the present."*

*F*iona lived her life to the full until sadly she died at the age of 38. She planned her funeral as carefully as she had planned her garden and left this message for us in the service of 'Celebration of her life':

"I want all my family and friends to know that I love them very much, and that because of their love and care, my life has been one in which the sadness has been far outweighed by the happiness and joy."

Fiona was and remains an inspiration to us all.

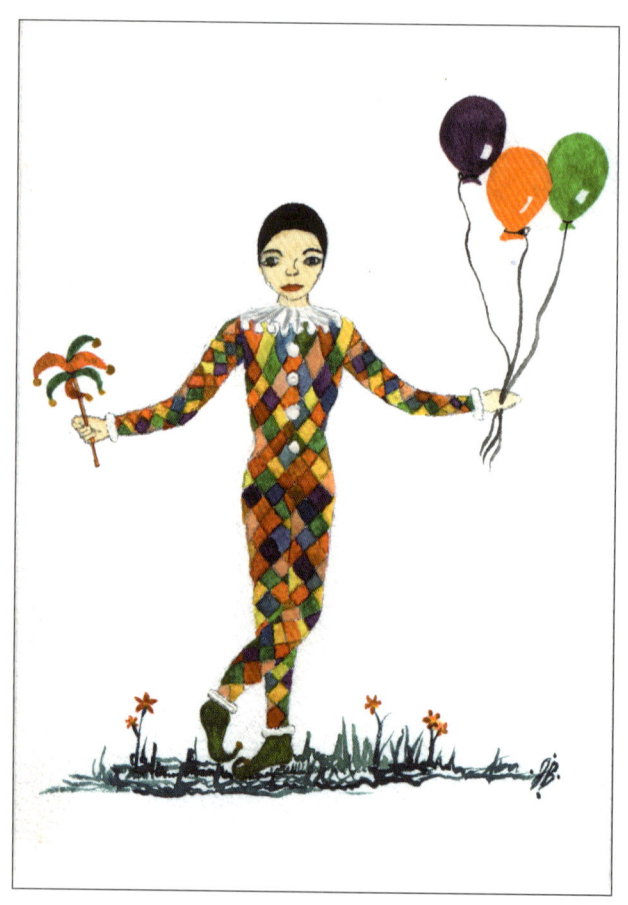

"Harlequin"

*H*ere, Now
I will not live in fear
But in joy for each day's turning.
For this the earth in all its beauty,
These are my friends with all their love,
And this is my life.
Here.
Now.

Fiona ~ after visiting the Bristol Centre

After Keith ~ from Clarissa

Just before Keith became very ill, we talked excitedly about making a trip to New Zealand to see the beautiful landscapes which were being used as a backdrop to a film of Tolkien's 'The Lord of the Rings', our favourite book. Sadly, it was a journey that we wouldn't make together. But I read to Keith from 'The Lord of the Rings' the night before he died, and I had opened it to read to him when he took his last breaths and passed on to some other place.

After Keith's funeral I decided to go to New Zealand alone. And it is truly beautiful. I did what Keith and I would have done together ~ walked on deserted beaches, sat by waterfalls or on the shores of turquoise lakes, trekked through rainforest, across glaciers, over strange moonscapes of geothermal activity, and imagined the journey that Frodo and his loyal servant Sam made to destroy the One Ring and banish the forces of evil from Middle Earth.

Later that year, on the exact anniversary of Keith's death *(19th December)*, 'The Fellowship of the Ring', the first part of the film of 'The Lord of the Rings', was released in England. My parents and I went to Leicester Square to see the first screening, and we remembered Keith as we were inspired by the characters and cinematography.

Early in the story Frodo discovers he is in possession of the evil and all-consuming Ring, and that the Dark Lord Sauron is looking for it. He exclaims to the wizard Gandalf that he wishes that it had not happened in his time. Gandalf wisely answers that so do all who live to see such times. But, he says, that is not for them to decide ~ all we have to decide is what to do with the time that is given us.

Keith made full use of the too short time given him, especially through his music teaching when he shared the joy of making music with everyone, whether they thought they were musical or not. I called Keith my angel-eyes. In his eyes I saw his generosity, enthusiasm, support and love, and I am thankful for the nine special years of life and love we shared together. When I realised that the film of our favourite story was to come out exactly a year to the day when Keith died, I felt that he was watching over me and I believe that in some way he always will.

Support Groups

"Friendship is born at the moment
when one person says to another ~
'What! You too? ~ I thought I was the only one'."
C. S. Lewis

*I*f you have cancer, one of the most helpful things you can do, in our opinion, is to make contact with someone else who has or has had cancer. In our experience we see that this indeed lightens the load. Within a group, there may be many people who are able to contribute to your recovery by sharing their knowledge and offering you friendship and support.

*T*he husband of one of our members expressed surprise when his wife felt the need to belong to a group. She had the support of a very close-knit family, who were initially a little disappointed that she felt she needed outside help. Later they understood and were happy that she'd found our Centre.

Treatments

"Instead of your treatment becoming a way of life,
your way of life becomes your treatment."

Sophie Barnes

"The cure of the part should not be attempted without treatment of the whole, and also no attempt should be made to cure the body without the soul, and therefore if the head and body are to be well you must begin by using the mind: that is the first thing ~ for this is the great error of our day in the treatment of the human body, that physicians separate the soul from the body."

Plato c427 BC.

*T*he wealth of complementary therapies now available can be quite overwhelming ~ and also expensive. It could be useful to contact your local Centre *(or our Centre if there isn't one in your area)* to see what is available free of charge, before launching into expensive treatments. Narrow down your choices. People quickly find therapists they warm to and others that they don't. Very often the choice is determined by the therapists themselves. It is important to find someone you feel comfortable with. As with all social interactions, it's a two-way arrangement. Our needs are different.

Some of our members highly recommend asking for a second opinion. Several have attended the Royal Marsden Hospital for this. Others feel that this implies lack of faith in their own consultant.

It is important to find what is 'right' for you. Fiona said that she hadn't been drawn to Counselling herself, but she acknowledged that others would find it beneficial. Keith based his approach on Vibrational therapies. But it isn't everyone who discusses Heisenberg's Uncertainty Principle with their Consultant!

Who to Contact

Your local Cancer Help Centre is a good place to start ~
or any of the following if there is no Centre
close to where you live.

Bristol Cancer Help Centre
Grove House
Cornwallis Street
Clifton
Bristol BS8 4PG
Telephone: 0117 980 9505/9500
www.bristolcancerhelp.org

Cambridge Cancer Help Centre
1a, Stockwell Street
off Mill Road
Cambridge CB1 3ND
Telephone: 01223 566151
(Tue/Wed 10am - 1pm)
www.cambridgecancerhelp.org

Cancerlink
Freephone support link
Telephone: 0808 808 0000
or 020 7833 2818
www.cancerlink org
Will listen to your concerns and put you in touch with the right support for you.

BACUP *(for medical advice)*
Will also help you to find a local group.
Telephone: 0800 181199

British Association of Nutritional Therapists (BANT)
www.bant.org.uk

Macmillan Cancer Relief
Telephone: 0845 601 6161
www.macmillan.org.uk

British Homeopathic Association
27a, Devonshire Street
London W1N 1RJ
Telephone: 020 7935 2163 *(1.30 –5pm)*
www.nhsconfed.net/bha

British Complementary Medicine Association (BCMA)
249, Fosse Road South
Leicester LE3 1AE
Telephone: 0116 282 5511
An umbrella organisation that holds a register of practitioners and produces a guide and a code of conduct for practitioners.

British Hypnotherapy Association
67, Upper Berkeley Street
London W1H 7 DH
Telephone: 020 7723 4443

Institute of Complementary Medicine
PO Box 194
London SE16 1QZ
Telephone: 020 7237 5165
(Mon.-Fri10am-2.30pm)
www.icmedicine.co.uk
Will help you to find a local therapist.

Books

We have an extensive library at our Centre. These are some of the books that are popular with our members.

We also have many useful relaxation tapes, CDs and videos.

The video produced by Bristol CHC is an excellent introduction to a spiritual approach. It can be obtained from Bristol for £25, which is refundable if you subsequently attend one of their courses.

Penny Brohn *Gentle Giants* and *The Bristol Programme*

Ayn W Cates *Consider this...*

Jenny Cole *Journeys (with a Cancer)*

Dr Rosy Daniel *Healing Foods*

Louise L Hay *You can heal your life*

William Johnston *Silent Music*

Elizabeth Kübler-Ross *On Death and Dying*

Lawrence LeShan *Cancer As a Turning Point* and *How to Meditate*

Paul Martin *The Sickening Mind*

Ainslie Meares *Let's be Human* and *The Wealth Within*

Iain Pearce *The Holistic Approach to Cancer*

S. Rippon *The Bristol Recipe Book*

Bernie Siegal *Love, Medicine and Miracles*

Carl Simonton *Getting Well Again*

Sandra Steingraber *Living Downstream*

Where next?

Ann's report at this year's AGM ended with the following ~

The Reverend Martin Luther King, on 28th August 1963 said 'I Have a Dream'. So I'm telling the Universe, as we are recommended to do, by those who believe it's the right thing to do, that although this Centre is a brilliant place, absolutely full of remarkable and courageous people, my dream is that one day we will own our own Centre, that it will be a peaceful, calm place ~ an oasis, and a continuing 'Shining Light', as it has recently been described.

Then all will be well.

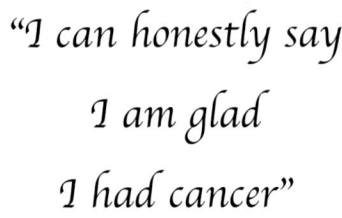

"I can honestly say
I am glad
I had cancer"

Marilyn Barnes